MAKE IT HAPPEN

WITHDRAWN
UTSA LIBRARIES

ACHE Management Series Editorial Board

Joseph J. Gilene, FACHE, Chairman
Quorum Health Resources

Mark C. Brown, FACHE
Lake City Medical Center-Mayo Health System

Robin B. Brown Jr., FACHE
Scripps Green Hospital

Frank A. Corvino, FACHE
Greenwich Hospital

Terence T. Cunningham III, FACHE
Shriners Hospital for Children

David A. Disbrow, FACHE
Ohio Cardiac Thoracic and Vascular Surgeons

Kent R. Helwig, FACHE
UT Southwestern Medical Center

Natalie D. Lamberton
Rio Rancho Medical Center

Trudy L. Land, FACHE
Executive Health Services

Greg Napps, FACHE
Bon Secours St. Mary's Hospital

James J. Sapienza, FACHE
MultiCare Health System

Arthur S. Shorr, FACHE
Arthur S. Shorr & Associates Inc.

Leticia W. Towns, FACHE
Regional Medical Center at Memphis

MAKE IT HAPPEN

EFFECTIVE EXECUTION IN HEALTHCARE LEADERSHIP

DANIEL B. MCLAUGHLIN

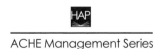

ACHE Management Series

Your board, staff, or clients may also benefit from this book's insight. For more information on quantity discounts, contact the Health Administration Press Marketing Manager at (312) 424–9470.

This publication is intended to provide accurate and authoritative information in regard to the subject matter covered. It is sold, or otherwise provided, with the understanding that the publisher is not engaged in rendering professional services. If professional advice or other expert assistance is required, the services of a competent professional should be sought.

The statements and opinions contained in this book are strictly those of the authors and do not represent the official positions of the American College of Healthcare Executives or the Foundation of the American College of Healthcare Executives.

Copyright © 2011 by the Foundation of the American College of Healthcare Executives. Printed in the United States of America. All rights reserved. This book or parts thereof may not be reproduced in any form without written permission of the publisher.

15   14   13   12   11   5   4   3   2   1

Library of Congress Cataloging-in-Publication Data

McLaughlin, Daniel B., 1945-
    Make it happen : effective execution in healthcare leadership/Daniel B. McLaughlin.
        p. ; cm.
Includes bibliographical references and index.
ISBN 978-1-56793-365-9 (alk. paper)
1. Health services administration. 2. Leadership. I. Title.
[DNLM: 1. Health Services Administration. 2. Leadership. W 84 AA1]
RA971.M4337 2011
362.1068--dc22
2010028820

The paper used in this publication meets the minimum requirements of American National Standard for Information Sciences—Permanence of Paper for Printed Library Materials, ANSI Z39.48-1984.∞™

Acquisitions editor: Janet Davis; Project manager: Eduard Avis; Cover designer: Marisa Jackson; Layout: Putman Productions, LLC

Found an error or a typo? We want to know! Please e-mail it to hap1@ache.org, and put "Book Error" in the subject line.

For photocopying and copyright information, please contact Copyright Clearance Center at www.copyright.com or at (978) 750–8400.

Health Administration Press
A division of the Foundation of the American
    College of Healthcare Executives
One North Franklin Street, Suite 1700
Chicago, IL 60606–3529
(312) 424–2800

Library
University of Texas
at San Antonio

To my wife, Sharon, and daughters, Kelly and Katie

Brief Contents

Detailed Contents

Preface

THIS BOOK IS about execution—how to design effective strategy, implement it, and make sure it works. It is based on the best practices of leading healthcare delivery systems, systems of execution outside of healthcare, and research results from both the business and healthcare literature.

I had the privilege of working for 30 years as an administrator for Hennepin County Medical Center (HCMC) in Minneapolis, Minnesota, including 8 years as CEO. I thought I was pretty good at getting things done when I was running a healthcare system, but I realize now that I could have been better. The challenge of execution was ever present in those years, but it has become even more intense today.

Fortunately, the last 30 years have seen the development of many new tools and approaches to improve execution in complex and rapidly changing environments. These tools are developed and spread through research and publication of books like this one, integration into higher education management curriculums, deployment by consultants, and adoption by progressive healthcare and business organizations.

I am glad Health Administration Press is publishing this book, because the company has a history of publishing research-based books for the healthcare administration field. Basic research and understanding underlie all such books. Next come applied research and concomitant publications that demonstrate how this fundamental science can be applied to solve real-world problems in areas such as strategy, project management, culture, and leadership. Many of these resources are the basis for the core elements of the chapters in this book, and I encourage readers to explore these publications to gain a greater understanding of these fundamental principles.

Because I read many business books and publications during my administrative career, I have crafted this book to contain elements I always thought were useful:

- A general overview of topics and references and resources that enabled me to learn more
- Enough detail so readers can try some of the tools or approaches in the book
- Stories about how the principles have been applied in actual practice by leading organizations
- I've also included web links, resources, and videos on the use of software mentioned in this book in an online Book Companion, which you can access at ache.org/books/execution.

When writing this book I was tempted to add many topics that would help, in some ways, to clarify some of the main points in the book. However, I finally felt this was too distracting and decided to focus in depth on what I consider the key elements of an integrated system for execution. For this reason, I did not touch on the following topics, even though they all clearly influence execution in a number of ways: finance and financial management, disruptive employees, negotiation and legal issues, marketing, structured innovation, human resources talent management, and personal time management. Readers are encouraged to access the many books on these topics available from Health Administration Press.

The Center for Health and Medical Affairs is part of the Opus College of Business at the University of St. Thomas, which is located in both Minneapolis and St. Paul, Minnesota. During its 20 years, the center has developed a broad array of healthcare management training programs, including a nationally accredited healthcare MBA program, a physician leadership college with over 200 graduates, and many other healthcare professional development programs. Over the years we have worked with all the major healthcare delivery systems in the upper Midwest to deliver custom programs to their staff and physicians. Therefore, most of the examples of best practices in this book come from organizations located in the upper Midwest. However, I was chair of the National Association of Public Hospitals and still have many hospital executive colleagues throughout the country who share their stories of execution challenges with me. Based on this, I believe the principles contained in this book are applicable to any geographic area. I also am confident that these tools can be applied in both large integrated systems and relatively small medical practices.

As I said, I could have better executed my strategies during my administrative career had I known what I know now. However, I have one small project that I did do well, and I still get to monitor its performance data. As an associate administrator at HCMC I was charged with sizing and then managing the construction of a large parking ramp for our employees. This was complex planning, as the Metrodome was being constructed next door (where the Vikings play), so I had to account for many diverse variables. I used the scenario planning technique described in Chapter 4 of this book along with some other quantitative decision tools and determined a peak need for this ramp of 850 spaces at 3:00 p.m. on weekdays. I still get my personal healthcare from HCMC, and if I have an appointment at about that time I drive to the top of the ramp to see how close it is to being full. So far the prediction is still pretty accurate—even after 30 years.

Hopefully you too will be able to use the tools in this book to execute strategies that last 30 years.

—Dan McLaughlin

CHAPTER 1

Introduction: The Need for Effective Execution in Healthcare

IN 2001 THE Institute of Medicine published *Crossing the Quality Chasm*. This seminal work identified the chasm between what is known about providing high-quality healthcare and what was actually being delivered. Unfortunately, this chasm remains open. This book provides healthcare organizations with a system for the effective execution of high-quality, cost-effective care.

The failure to execute is a common problem in many organizations, but especially in healthcare. The barriers to effective execution are well understood and include an incredibly complex system, splintered leadership, strategies that vacillate between financial goals and patient care, and no external pressure strong enough to force change.

However, external pressures that will force change in the system continue to build. Unsustainable cost growth and uneven quality cannot continue. In response to many of these trends Congress enacted the Patient Protection and Affordable Care Act of 2010, which is the largest change in health policy in the United States since the inception of Medicare. It will significantly change the system through numerous features that reward performance and value but penalize those providers who are unwilling to change. In the face of this rapidly changing environment, many progressive healthcare delivery organizations are now seeking a path to become "high performance" health systems.

The Commonwealth Fund Commission defines a high performance health system as "one that helps everyone, to the extent possible, lead longer, healthier, and more productive lives. To achieve such a system, four core goals must be met: access to care for all; safe, high-quality care; efficient, high-value care; and continuous innovation and improvement" (The Commonwealth Fund Commission on a High Performance Health System 2007).

To achieve this status, many organizations will have to change dramatically. They will need to become true "health systems," as opposed to facilities that focus on curing the sick. In addition, value-based purchasing and bending the cost curve will be parts of this new competitive environment, and organizations will need to find ways to meet these marketplace and regulatory demands. Healthcare organizations that can develop and effectively execute their plans will thrive, while those that cannot will struggle and eventually be absorbed by their more effective competitors.

Fortunately, the systems that support the effective execution of strategy are well known and practiced by many of America's most successful corporations. This book translates these systems to the healthcare environment and details their use by leading healthcare delivery organizations.

THE EMERGING IMPORTANCE OF EXECUTION IN HEALTHCARE

During the first 60 years of the twentieth century, the clinical and business aspects of healthcare were led by physicians because both clinical technology and the financial aspects of healthcare were relatively simple. However, clinical technology began to expand rapidly during World War II, and the Great Society programs of the 1960s (Medicare and Medicaid) expanded the scope and complexity of healthcare financing. During these years physicians began to focus on clinical issues and often left the business functions to specialists—frequently individuals with MHAs or MBAs. However, this separation of duties is now coming to a close as society is demanding a more efficient and integrated healthcare system (see Exhibit 1.1). The successful future healthcare organization will focus on quality, patient safety, financial stewardship, and physician, patient, and employee satisfaction.

Structures for the delivery of care will change as more and more physicians join hospitals or larger clinics to achieve financial stability. The success of these new complex organizations will hinge on their ability to use disciplined management tools to plan, execute, and monitor their organization's performance.

A SYSTEM FOR EXECUTION IN HEALTHCARE

This book provides a comprehensive system for effective execution in the healthcare environment. It is based on best practices from leading healthcare

Exhibit 1.1
Changing
Emphasis in
Healthcare

1930s to 1960s—Emphasis on New Clinical Breakthroughs

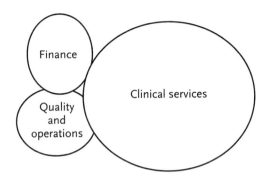

1960s to 2010—Emphasis on New Funding Resources and Growth

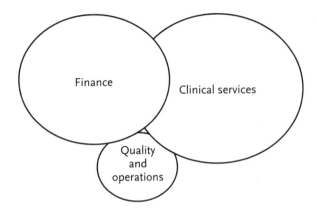

The Future—Emphasis on Quality and Value

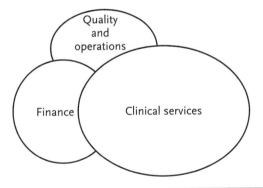

organizations, state-of-the-art approaches to execution in other industries, and the author's (and his university colleagues') experiences in providing professional development training to healthcare leaders. It has four major sections: strategy, tools, people, and systems.

I. Strategy—Developing a Focused Strategic Plan

Although this book is not primarily about strategy development, a poorly conceived plan is difficult to execute effectively. (In some cases, there is no plan at all.) Therefore, the fundamentals and contemporary concepts of strategic planning are reviewed here with an emphasis on effective approaches used by leading healthcare organizations.

The use of large databases as an aid to planning is just emerging in healthcare. This book explores the concepts of the business intelligence approach—including data warehousing, data mining, and benchmarking—which can be extremely useful in creating and monitoring plans. Finally, the emerging strategic plan can be made more robust and tested for flexibility through the use of scenario analysis.

II. Tools—Contemporary Business Methods of Execution

The use of business tools to execute change is a major focus of this book. The balanced scorecard has been used by corporations for many years to move strategy to action, and now leading healthcare organizations also use it. Project management is the basic tool of execution, and the formal project management methodology as promulgated by the PMI (Project Management Institute) will be detailed. This also includes the use of the project management office to monitor and support multiple simultaneous projects. Modifications to the formal project management system and the implementation of clinical innovations will be explored as well.

Once performance gains have been achieved, an organization needs to sustain these gains by embedding the changes it has made. Although most strategies are executed by individuals, many new powerful, automated tools support change reinforcement. The use of computerized business rules and performance monitoring to support execution will be outlined.

III. People—Leading Individuals and Organization for Effective Change

Even the most sophisticated use of business tools will fail to achieve desired organizational results if the people in an organization are not led well and do not feel engaged. This section of the book explores these challenges. Employee engagement and organizational culture can either impede or support effective execution; contemporary approaches will be reviewed with a special emphasis on practical approaches to improving both. An organization's structure and compensation systems are also important factors in effective execution; best practices in these areas will be detailed.

The adaptive leadership model developed by Dr. Ron Heifetz (Heifetz and Linsky 2002) is well suited to the healthcare environment and has been used effectively by the 150+ graduates of University of St. Thomas's Physician Leadership College. The key elements of adaptive leadership will be explored with detailed examples.

IV. Systems—An Integrated System for Execution in Healthcare

The final section ties all the elements together—strategy, tools, and people—into a comprehensive system for execution.

The Malcolm Baldrige National Quality Award is a coveted honor given to only one or two healthcare organizations each year. The execution system detailed in this book can be a key component of an organization's journey to achieving many of the goals of the Baldrige Award.

A high performance healthcare system is a challenge to achieve and maintain. However, effective execution can make this journey easier, more satisfying, and longer lasting.

HOW THE CHAPTERS ARE ORGANIZED

Most of the chapters in this book are organized into four major sections:

- **State of the art**—A description of best practices in the uses of the chapter's business tool or leadership approach
- **Notes from the field**—Examples from leading healthcare organizations on the use of the business tool, with strong connections to the state of the art
- **Vincent Valley Healthcare System (VVH)**[1]—A fictional but realistic healthcare system featured to illustrate the use of these business tools and people skills (Because much of this book contains tools and concepts that are just beginning to be used in healthcare, no one existing organization can be used to demonstrate the full breadth of these tools' power—hence the use of VVH. In addition, stories are powerful learning tools and help embed concepts more easily than formal business narratives. It is hoped readers can translate VVH's use of these skills and tools to their own organizations.)
- **Summary**—Key issues and lessons from the chapter

COMPANION TEXTBOOK

Healthcare Operations Management[2] is a complementary resource to this book. Whereas this book is focused on effectively executing an organization's strategy, *Healthcare Operations Management* is focused on maintaining the gains and making continuous improvements in ongoing operations. It also contains a comprehensive approach to unique operational challenges, such as Lean Six Sigma for process improvement, scheduling optimization, and supply change management.

NOTES

1. VVH is located in a Midwestern city of 1.5 million people. It has 3,000 employees, operates 350 inpatient beds, and has a medical staff of 450 physicians. In addition, VVH operates nine clinics staffed by physicians who are employees of the system. VVH has two major competitor hospitals, and a number of surgeons from all three hospitals recently joined together to set up an independent ambulatory surgery center.

2. *Healthcare Operations Management*, McLaughlin and Hays, Health Administration Press, 2008, 466 pages.

SECTION I

STRATEGY

Do not repeat the tactics which have gained you one victory, but let your methods be regulated by the infinite variety of circumstances.

Sun Tzu, Chinese military strategist, c. 490 BC

CHAPTER 2

Developing Strategic Focus

ORGANIZATIONS THAT EXECUTE effectively create and maintain a focused and disciplined strategic plan. Although this book is not primarily about strategic planning, a review of basic planning concepts and their use by leading healthcare organizations will support the execution tools detailed in the remainder of the book.

This chapter provides

- a rationale for a strong strategic plan,
- alternative approaches to strategic planning and an introduction to scenario planning—envisioning alternative futures, and
- a model for healthcare strategic planning today.

STATE OF THE ART

Rationale for Strategic Planning

Strategic planning originated with early military organizations—many historic battle victories can be attributed to a strategic plan. In the 1940s and 1950s, budgeting and planning became part of progressive business operations. These tools developed into the more sophisticated planning systems formed in the 1960s and still in use today.

Many healthcare organizations, particularly hospitals, followed these models. The advent of Medicare and the Great Society programs in the 1960s injected substantial new money into the healthcare system. As a result, strategic planning during the period from 1970 to 1990 focused on growth and facilities expansion. A comprehensive strategic plan was required to accurately determine the size of new facilities and in some cases support a Certificate of Need application. As the possibility of health reform loomed in the early 1990s, the focus of strategic planning changed to developing managed care capabilities and strengthening physician relationships. However, the failure of the Clinton Health Plan in 1994 precipitated a shift in focus toward the consumer.

Each of these trends in strategic planning built upon its predecessor so that most formal healthcare strategic plans today contain all of these elements. The current emphasis is on value—a combination of costs, quality, and safety—in healthcare delivery.

Some have argued that because of the dynamics of the healthcare environment, formal strategic planning systems are not necessary. This criticism focuses on the complex, slow, and expensive bureaucratic processes that frequently generate plans that are not connected to daily operations. However, without a strategic plan an organization may not anticipate major shifts in technology, markets, patient preferences, competition, or regulatory changes. It also risks not developing core competencies needed for long-term sustainability (Baldrige National Quality Program 2010, p. 10).

Models of Strategic Planning

Although many large healthcare organizations use a fairly traditional model as outlined by Zuckerman (discussed later in the chapter), Mintzberg (Mintzberg, Ahlstrand, and Lampel 1998) provides a useful overview of the multiple approaches many organizations have used to create effective strategic plans. He calls them "schools" to signify the breadth of each approach.

The first and oldest is the *Design School* of planning. This planning approach seeks to find an optimal fit between an organization's internal capabilities and its external possibilities. The core tool of this approach is the SWOT analysis, in which an organization determines its Strengths, Weaknesses, Opportunities, and Threats and then crafts a strategy to maximize the Strengths and Opportunities and minimize the Weaknesses and Threats. Although this methodology is still widely used, it does not take advantage of other components of strategy developments such as incremental and emergent strategy formulation and the influence of structure on strategy (see Chapter 9).

The *Planning School* builds on the Design School concept by taking a more formal approach to the strategic planning process. This process includes distinct steps, checklists, forms, and timelines. The process is owned by the CEO and managed by staff planners. The final strategies are fully developed, with expected outcomes, timelines, and budgets. Although many

Exhibit 2.1
The Boston
Consulting
Group Growth-
Share Matrix

	Growth Potential		
	Star	Problem child	
	Cash cow	Dog	

Current Market Share

Source: The Boston Consulting Group, Boston, MA. Used with permission.

organizations used this system throughout the latter part of the twentieth century, many failures occurred. Academics who dissected these failures determined a number of causes, such as a disconnect between staff ownership of the process and operations, a focus on mergers and acquisitions rather than on core operations, a lack of understanding of an organization's culture, and an inability to respond effectively to a rapidly changing environment.

The *Positioning School* takes a different approach. Proponents of this school examine the content of strategic plans and determine an optimal mix of "positions" to take to achieve an organization's goals. The most famous of these positioning strategies was promulgated by The Boston Consulting Group growth-share matrix (see Exhibit 2.1) (Mintzberg et al. 1998, p. 95).

Products or services with high market share and slow growth are "cash cows," while those with low market share and slow growth are "dogs." Low market share, high growth products are "problem children" that must be managed carefully, and high share, high growth products are "stars." According to Mintzberg and colleagues (1998, p. 96), a well-balanced portfolio strategy has

- "stars," whose high share and high growth ensure future profitability;
- "cash cows" that supply funds for future growth;
- "problem children" that should be converted into "stars" with added funds and attention; and
- "dogs," which should be eliminated or sold.

Exhibit 2.2 depicts a balanced portfolio for an integrated health system. The strategic initiatives taken to balance this portfolio are in italics. Although useful as a part of the strategic planning process, the Positioning School by itself cannot be used to develop a comprehensive strategic plan.

The *Learning School* is a significantly different approach to strategic planning, as it moves much of the energy from the executive suite to the front

Exhibit 2.2
Growth-Share
Matrix for an
Integrated
Healthcare
Delivery System

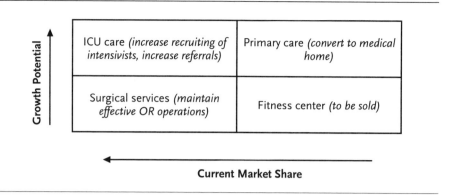

lines of the organization. It is based on the recognition that most organizations operate in a complex and unpredictable environment. Therefore, strategy formulation takes the form of continuous learning and change.

This methodology contends that strategies grow like weeds from throughout the organization and "can take root in all kinds of places, virtually anywhere people have the capacity and the resources to support that capacity" (Mintzberg 1998, p. 196). These grassroots strategies become organizational when they grow large enough and collective enough to pervade the organization. This process may be conscious but need not be. However, it is incumbent on organizational leaders to recognize these emergent strategies and integrate them into whatever formal strategic planning process is in place.

The Learning School approach is frequently seen in clinical innovations (see Chapter 7). A physician may attend a conference, learn a new clinical treatment approach, begin to use it, and then ask an organizational leader for more resources to fully implement this new tool. The well-managed organization does not view this event as a violation of the annual strategic planning process but anticipates and encourages this creative entrepreneurial energy.

Scenario Planning

In many ways, the traditional strategic plan assumes that the organization is operating in a stable environment, which rarely exists. However, by using scenario planning an organization can develop a rapid strategic response capability. Scenario planning is used in conjunction with strategic planning to develop possible futures. The organization's strategic plan is then tested against these scenarios to determine its robustness (ability to rapidly and effectively adjust). The process of scenario planning will be further detailed in Chapter 4, and culture will be explored in Chapter 10.

Healthcare Strategic Planning Today

In his book *Healthcare Strategic Planning*, Alan Zuckerman (2005) provides a useful template for a strategic planning system used by many leading healthcare organizations today. In this traditional model there are four phases: environmental assessment, organizational direction, strategy formulation, and implementation planning. Exhibit 2.3 provides an overview of this process.

Chapter 3 of this book details contemporary tools for internal and external analysis as part of the organizational assessment. Chapter 4 provides a framework for developing alternative futures and formulating an effective strategy. The remainder of this book outlines the business tools and people skills needed to effectively execute these strategies.

NOTES FROM THE FIELD

HealthPartners

HealthPartners is an integrated healthcare system that includes a large medical group, three hospitals, and a health plan with over 1.2 million members (see appendix for more detail).

HealthPartners uses many of the traditional elements of the Design and Planning schools as described by Zuckerman (2005). It has a centralized strategic planning process but key strategies, tactics, and execution are handled by the operating units and aligned with the overall plan. It operates on a three-year planning cycle with four dimensions: people, health, experience, and stewardship. Each dimension has a council with director-level staff as members. Each council develops both high level and departmental goals for each year.

Success for each dimension at HealthPartners is described as:

People—A highly engaged and committed workforce
Health—Improved health for our patients, members, and community
Experience—Deliver an exceptional experience that customers want and deserve at an affordable cost
Stewardship—Deliver greater value, growth, and financial results

The corporate goals are then translated into more specific departmental goals and summarized in a strategic matrix (Exhibit 2.4).

Exhibit 2.3 Strategic Planning Process

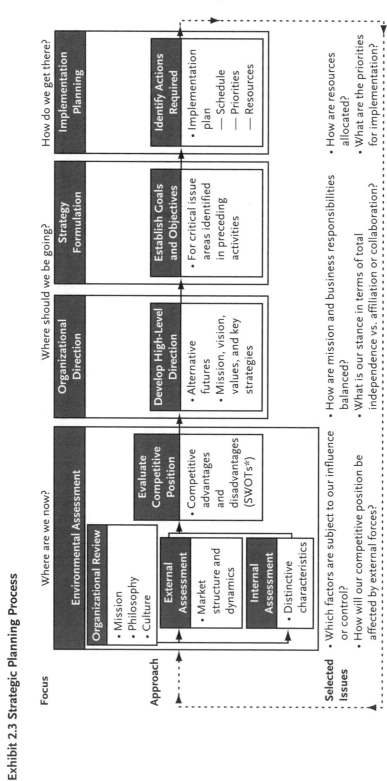

*SWOTs = strengths, weaknesses, opportunities, and threats.

© 2004 Health Strategies and Solutions, Inc.

Source: Zuckerman (2005, p. 7). Reprinted with permission.

Exhibit 2.4
HealthPartners
Strategy Matrix

	Corporate goals	How to get there	Specific departmental goals and metrics
People			
Healthcare			
Patient experience			
Stewardship			

Source: HealthPartners, Bloomington, MN. Used with permission.

Department-level metrics are tracked monthly and the results are sent to each council. Every six months, each council meets with the senior executive team to review progress and challenges that may need additional attention.

Twin Cities Orthopedics

In contrast to the large integrated system just discussed, Twin Cities Orthopedics (TCO) takes more of a Learning School approach to strategic planning. TCO is a single-specialty practice of 79 physicians, 74 of whom are orthopedic surgeons. It is a unique combination of many small practices into one large practice with a number of divisions (see Chapter 9 for more discussion on structure). The surgeon leaders of this group are not interested in complex, time-consuming systems of planning and devote only one meeting of their board to this activity per year.

However, the board has developed a strong relationship with the practice's administrative staff, and these individuals do much of the detailed planning. TCO's strategic initiatives are organized into three perspectives: service, collaboration, and financial results. Metrics in these areas are tracked and reported to the board monthly. A powerful aspect of this type of planning is TCO's ability to quickly adopt new technologies, change locations, or acquire other practices.

VINCENT VALLEY HEALTHCARE

Todd Stinson had been a three-term legislator before coming to work as the chief strategy officer at Vincent Valley Healthcare System (VVH). Before he was elected, he had earned a master's degree in health administration and worked for five years at two major health systems in Chicago. However, his father had been speaker of the state house of representatives and his dad's colleagues had recruited him back home to run for the legislature.

In 2008 he started to see the momentum rise for significant changes in the healthcare system. Rising costs, uneven quality, frequent errors, and public policy's growing role in shaping the system made the environment attractive for someone who wanted to help implement change. The healthcare reform bill passed in 2010 reinforced this need for change and provided a number of interesting opportunities for VVH. The system hired him to manage its legislative policy agenda at the state level and develop strategy to meet the community's needs and to take advantage of some of the new programs available under the Patient Protection and Affordable Care Act.

Because of rising costs in the system, Stinson knew that policymakers would eventually support an expansion of various Medicare and state-based experiments that were now starting to show results. He encouraged VVH's leaders to engage in similar initiatives in order to be prepared for the healthcare system of the future. He was particularly pleased to see that structures such as accountable care organizations (ACOs), the medical home, and bundled payment systems for hospital admissions were included in the new law.

Stinson provided a review of these possible new initiatives to the executive team of VVH as it kicked off its annual review and update of the organization's strategic plan. Susan Francis, the CEO, was positive and optimistic about new opportunities for VVH but shared her need to focus her time on governance changes under way in the system. Her message was, "After this plan is updated and we feel we have a robust strategy, we need to execute more effectively and quickly than we have in the past—particularly in light of significant reimbursement challenges and the need to engage our physicians and staff in new ways."

She also expressed concern that failed execution was dangerous and told the story of a graduate school classmate who had led a system similar to VVH. Over the past two years, he had poorly executed a major installation of an electronic health record system. This failed execution prompted physician unrest and significant operating losses and cost the executive his job. After relating this story, Francis again emphasized that execution was the key skill needed by the executive team and asked Bob Olson, the COO, to lead this new effort to improve execution.

The executive planning team examined its existing strategic plan by applying the SWOT methodology but focused much of its effort on the opportunities it felt were now available due to the successful experiments Stinson had reviewed. The discussion focused on many of the elements of these new initiatives, but the team felt VVH could succeed with a new

ACO-type structure, a medical home, and bundled payments for inpatient care. It asked Stinson to explore ways to partner with government and private payers to support these initiatives.

VVH organized its strategic plan into four perspectives:

- Patient care
- Operations
- People
- Financial support

The ACO and bundled payment initiatives were considered part of the operations perspective, while the medical home was more closely connected to the patient care perspective. The executive team felt these projects could be effectively executed within the existing VVH structure—particularly with the new execution tools Olson would soon be implementing.

The team also saw an opportunity for growth in the Tasker Foothills area. Although close to the VVH service area, the Foothills were home to many small practices that referred to four different systems and hospitals. Dr. Cynthia Andresen was a well-respected internist in the Foothills and was a classmate of Dr. Ira Moscone, the chief medical officer of VVH. At a recent alumni event, Andresen told Moscone that many of her colleagues in the Foothills area were anxious about succeeding in the challenging payment environment but did not want to give up their autonomy. Moscone proposed to the team that he explore new relationships with these practices with the eventual goal of creating a medical home initiative for the area.

The team agreed that the existing VVH strategic planning process would not work well for this project and suggested that Moscone work with these practices using the Learning School approach—that is, consistently take small steps that improve each practice every day. The next day Moscone called Andresen and asked if he could take her and some of her colleagues in the Foothills area out to dinner to discuss the possibility of using a portion of the VVH billing system to improve collection rates and cash flow. He also mentioned that demonstrations being developed around the medical home concept might pose new revenue opportunities.

SUMMARY

An organization that executes well has an effective strategic planning process. A strategic plan is the foundation for executing in a timely and cost-effective manner.

A number of approaches can be used to create an effective plan. The most traditional approach is a combination of the Design School, which uses SWOT analysis, and the Planning School, which includes a sophisticated and well-managed planning process. Most large integrated healthcare systems use this combination and implement it in four phases:

- Organizational assessment
- High level organizational goal setting
- Strategy development
- Implementation planning and monitoring

Most effective strategic plans also consider the positioning of various product lines within the market to assess their potential to fund and grow market share. The Positioning School takes a different, but complementary, approach by examining the content of strategic plans and determining an optimal mix of "positions" needed to achieve an organization's goals.

An alternative approach to strategic planning is the Learning School, in which small changes are continuously implemented and the sum of these changes constitutes the organization's strategic plan. The Learning School approach to planning is nimble and responds quickly to environmental changes. However, because it is difficult to use the Learning School approach in large organizations, these organizations instead use multiple future scenarios to test the robustness and agility of their strategic plans.

RESOURCES

Note: Internet links to these resources can be found in the Book Companion (www.ache.org/pubs/hap_companion/index_3.cfm) that accompanies this book.

The Centers for Medicare & Medicaid Services has implemented a number of demonstration projects in the following areas:

- ACOs are partially based on the Medicare Physician Group Practice Demonstration (www.cms.hhs.gov).
- Medical homes (www.aafp.org) demonstration is under way.
- Bundled payments are being tested by the Acute Care Episode (ACE) demonstration project (www.cms.hhs.gov).
- The Institute for Healthcare Improvement's "Hospital to Home" strategy (www.h2hquality.org) is designed to prevent unnecessary readmissions and optimize financial performance under bundled payments.

Internal and External Assessment Using Business Intelligence

A KEY COMPONENT of developing a strategic plan is a review of an organization's internal performance data and external benchmarks. This review will identify deviations from the current plan and reveal opportunities that are not readily apparent. An effective internal and benchmark analysis converts masses of data into useful knowledge. This knowledge serves as a platform for updating and refining an organization's strategic plan.

This section will explore current and advanced concepts of organizational assessment:

- Data sources for internal analysis
- Data warehousing
- Performance reporting
- Data mining
- External benchmarking

STATE OF THE ART

Data Sources for Internal Analysis

All contemporary organizations use automated systems to generate reports and, in fact, most information systems generate too many reports. This sea of data makes it challenging for the manager to find meaningful and actionable information. This section outlines basic tools for collecting, displaying, and reviewing data. Chapter 5—The Balanced Scorecard—builds on these techniques and outlines a method for connecting performance metrics to the strategic plan.

	Stage	Cumulative Capabilities
Exhibit 3.1 HIMSS Analytics EMR Adoption Model (summarized)	0	No ancillary computer systems installed (pharmacy, laboratory, radiology)
	1	All ancillaries installed
	2	Clinical data repository active, rudimentary clinical decision support, document imaging, connection to a health information exchange
	3	Nursing/clinical information (flow sheets), clinical decision support (drug/drug, drug/food, drug/lab), medical imaging access available
	4	Computerized practitioner order entry (CPOE), decision support of evidence-based medicine
	5	Closed loop medication administration
	6	Physician documentation (structured templates), full decision support, full access to imaging
	7	No paper, full EHR, data warehouse and analytical tools, external data sharing, full continuity of data into ED and ambulatory clinics

Source: HIMSS Analytics (2009). www.himssanalytics.org/docs/HA_EMRAM_Overview_ENG.pdf. Used with permission.

Since the advent of the electronic health record (EHR, also called electronic medical record [EMR]), sources of electronic data have been proliferating. The EHR is an addition to most organizations' financial, human resources, and unique departmental systems. The Healthcare Information and Management Systems Society (HIMSS) provides a useful scale to determine an organization's maturity in implementing EHRs[1] (see Exhibit 3.1).

Installing these systems is usually challenging and expensive. The databases created by clinical systems are large and complex and not easily accessed. However, they provide a unique and unprecedented view into the real core of healthcare operations—the delivery of clinical care.

This challenge has been addressed for a number of years by businesses outside of healthcare. *Business intelligence* (BI) is the term used for a new suite of information technology capabilities that helps organizations understand their current operations and plan for the future. The key components of BI include

- data warehousing,
- performance reporting, and
- data mining.

A classic example of the use of BI techniques has been demonstrated by Harrah's Casino. By having casino patrons swipe an electronic card to play the casino's games, the casino collects real-time information on an individual's wins and losses. This information is then moved to a data warehouse and mined.

Using this data, Harrah's staff discovered they could predict a "pain point" for every gambler's daily losses. Customers who exceeded this level seldom came back. In response, Harrah's implemented a real-time monitoring system (see the section on automated business rules in Chapter 9) and developed a protocol to follow when this type of customer comes close to his or her pain point. Instead of idly watching the gambler continue to lose money, a Harrah's employee approaches this individual and says, "I see you are having a rough day. I know you like our steakhouse. Here—I'd like to take you and your wife to dinner on us right now." What could have been a lost customer is turned into a loyal customer (Ayers 2007, p. 31).

Data Warehousing

Organizational leaders frequently ask seemingly simple questions of their information technology departments that actually require complex processing to answer. Nothing is more frustrating than to go through the organizational pain and financial cost of installing a new electronic health record system and then find out you cannot retrieve what seems to be the most mundane data. Yet this frequently occurs. This conundrum is due to the complex structure of today's operating systems, which are primarily designed to manage large data sets.

The solution to this problem is the data warehouse. A data warehouse is a separate, but connected, computer system designed for accurate data storage, performance reporting, and data mining. Data warehouses also usually contain data marts, which are smaller, subject-specific databases. Most database software today allows all data marts in an organization to be combined into a data warehouse. Exhibit 3.2 shows the relationship of the operating systems, the data warehouse, and online analytical tools.

The following are the key structural elements of an effective data warehouse:

- It is subject oriented and data are organized from the users' point of view.
- It is an integrated database that combines data from different sources and removes errors where possible.

Exhibit 3.2 A Data Warehouse Environment

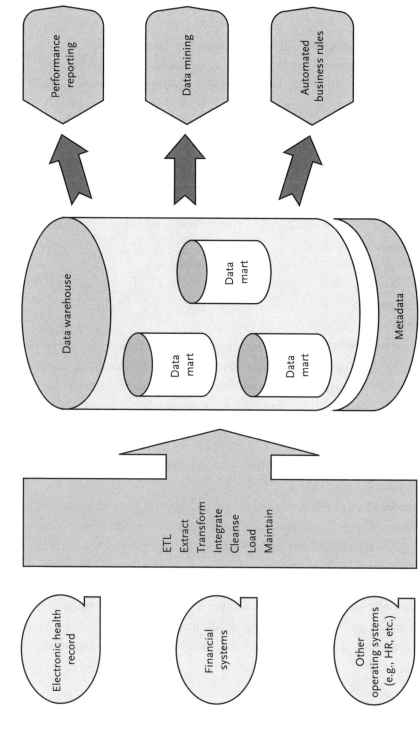

- It is time variant—each data element has an associated time.
- It is non-volatile—the data are static and do not change, and new data supplement, rather than replace, existing data.

Extract, Transform, and Load (ETL)

To create and update the warehouse, data are obtained from the operational systems and loaded into the data warehouse through an extract, transform, and load process abbreviated as ETL. In this process, data are extracted from the operating systems and transformed into a database format designed for analysis. Data elements are also integrated and connected with each other as needed.

An interesting challenge in creating a data warehouse is that approximately 10 percent of data entered by humans is wrong. The ETL process cleanses the data where possible to eliminate errors that can lead to misleading results in an analysis.

Data are extracted from the operating systems on varied schedules. In healthcare environments, many data marts are updated monthly (e.g., financial information), while others are updated daily (e.g., pharmacy information).

During ETL some additional processing may occur. Most health plans have large claims databases that they analyze in a data warehouse. During the ETL procedure, the plans use software that uses the diagnosis and treatment fields to categorize each claim into an episode of treatment group (ETG). The 600 ETGs are then used for subsequent analysis of provider behavior and costs.

Metadata

Metadata are also part of the warehouse; they are "data about the data." To effectively analyze the data in a warehouse, the user needs to understand data definitions, structure, and syntax. Practitioners who use healthcare data warehouses report that one of their primary challenges is reaching organizational agreement on what appear to be simple data definitions (e.g., a hospital discharge, a birth, a visit that is determined to be uncompensated, and many more).

Analysis

Once the data marts, data warehouse, and metadata are established, analytical software is used for performance reporting and data mining. In addition,

Exhibit 3.3
Comparison of
Operating
System to Data
Warehouse

Aspect	Transactional Data System	Data Warehouse
Data content	Current activities	Historical summary
Supports	Operational applications	Understanding of business area
Nature of changes to the data	Dynamic updating	Static until reloaded or refreshed
Usage	Predictable and repetitive	Analytical, ad hoc

automated business rules can be implemented; business rules systems will be described more fully in Chapter 9.

The differences between an operational system and a data warehouse are summarized in Exhibit 3.3.

Creating a useful data warehouse is a challenge for both the information technology department and the users. It is costly and requires skill to use properly. However, it is a powerful tool for developing, executing, and monitoring strategies.

Performance Reporting

To access data in the warehouse, analysts use software known as On Line Analytical Processing (OLAP) tools.

Analysts using OLAP tools do four types of processing:

1. **Categorical analysis** is a static analysis of historical data. Examples include number of visits to the emergency department per month and number of full-time equivalents (FTEs) in the pharmacy department.
2. **Exegetical analysis**[2] is also based on historical data, but the online reports include the capability to "drill down" into the data by clicking on report elements. See Exhibit 3.4 for an example of a drill-down report for an expense budget.
3. **Contemplative analysis** allows a user to change a single value in interlinked data to determine its effect. For example, a financial report could be constructed from data in the warehouse and various revenue scenarios could be modeled.
4. **Formulaic analysis** expands contemplative analysis to allow changes to multiple variables (Turban et al. 2008, p. 94).

Exhibit 3.4
Drill-Down
Reporting

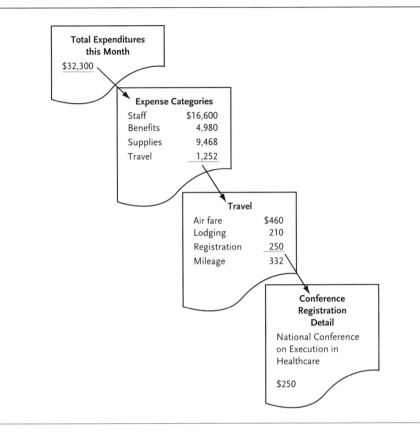

Most performance reporting in healthcare resides in four domains:

- Finance
- Patient/customer experience
- Clinical care
- Workforce

Because many of the interesting questions managers ask cross these domains, it is critical that the construction of the data warehouse allow reporting across all domains. For example, an analyst might want to know the clinical outcomes and cost for a specific Diagnosis Related Group (DRG) for a specific physician.

Graphical Data Displays

Graphical displays are a key ingredient of OLAP software and help the user understand data relationships and changes over time. The following types of graphs are often used in dashboards and scorecards.

Exhibit 3.5 Bar and Column Charts

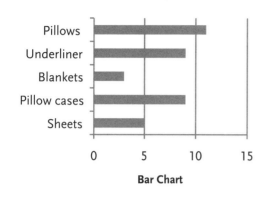

Bar Chart

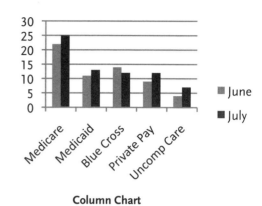

Column Chart

**Exhibit 3.6
Fuel Gauge
Indicator**

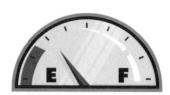

**Exhibit 3.7
Line Chart**

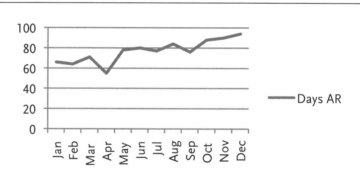

Bar charts illustrate comparisons among individual items. Column charts are useful for showing data changes over a certain period and for illustrating comparisons among items (Exhibit 3.5).

Because dashboards are now widely used, the classic fuel gauge is making a comeback and is used to indicate the performance of individual metrics (see Exhibit 3.6).

Line charts can display continuous data over time, set against a common scale, and are therefore ideal for showing trends in data at equal intervals (Exhibit 3.7).

Exhibit 3.8
Pie Chart

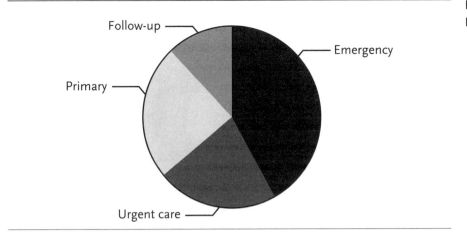

Exhibit 3.9
Scatter Chart
with Linear
Regression Line

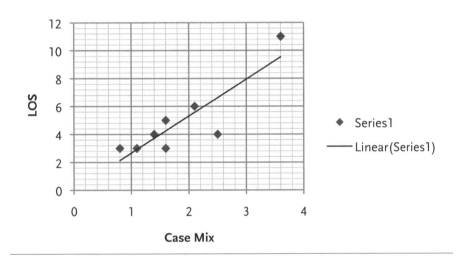

Pie charts show the size of items in one data series, proportional to the sum of the items. The data points in a pie chart are displayed as actual data or a percentage of the whole pie (Exhibit 3.8).

Area charts emphasize the magnitude of change over time and can be used to draw attention to the total value across a trend.

Scatter charts show the relationships among the numeric values in several data series, or they plot two groups of numbers as one series of x-y coordinates. In addition, most charting software enables the user to draw a regression line to indicate correlations in the data (see Exhibit 3.9).

More complex displays are also available but should be used with caution, as they are not easily understood by the infrequent viewer. Like a pie chart, a *doughnut chart* (Exhibit 3.10) shows the relationship of parts to a whole, but it can contain more than one data series. *Radar charts* (Exhibit 3.11) compare

Exhibit 3.10
Doughnut Chart

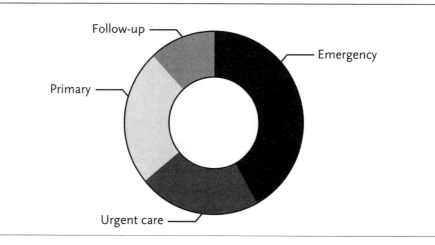

Exhibit 3.11
Radar Chart

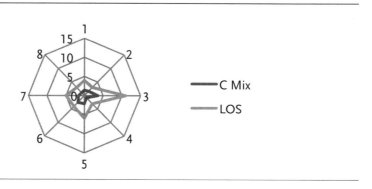

Exhibit 3.12
Surface Chart

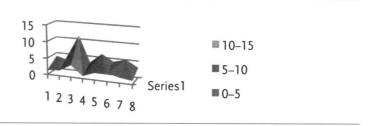

the aggregate values of several data series. A *surface chart* (Exhibit 3.12) is useful for finding optimal combinations between two sets of data. As in a topographic map, colors and patterns indicate areas that are in the same range of values.

A relatively new display is the *Sparkline*, popularized by Edward Tufte (whom many consider the grand master of information display). It is essentially a small line chart reduced to show the trend or relationship without axes and labels. This simplification helps clearly convey important information. Sparklines can be embedded in other displays and are particularly powerful when they are embedded in text displays (see Exhibit 3.13).

Exhibit 3.13 Inpatient Census—Medical Surgical Units, Monthly Average with Sparklines

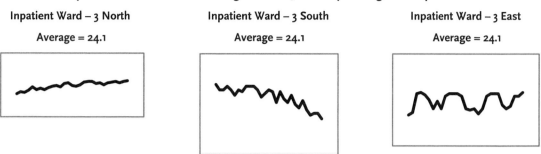

Note that the single number (Monthly Average) is misleading and the Sparkline provides deeper information.

Predictive Analysis

Another feature of most OLAP software is the ability to do predictive analysis. The basis for this capability is statistical methods that are beyond the scope of this book. However, when used correctly, predictive analysis can be helpful in optimizing operations and strategic performance. Some of the analytical techniques commonly used are

- moving averages,
- exponential smoothing,
- seasonal and cyclical modeling,
- linear regression, and
- autoregressive integrated moving average models (ARIMA).

For a fuller explanation, refer to *Healthcare Operations Management*, Chapter 13: Supply Chain Management.

Data Mining

Almost all performance reporting is directed by users and is focused on understanding a specific business or clinical issue. However, many organizations also use data mining tools to discover information in their data that is not readily apparent. Data mining is the process of extracting non-trivial, previously unknown, and potentially useful information from large databases.

Because of the recent installation of EHRs, most BI applications in healthcare today are based on performance reporting—understanding basic questions about an organization's actual functioning. Here are some example questions:

- Which doctors utilize imaging the most?
- What is the clinical difference in the outcomes of using two separate classes of drugs for patients with a similar condition?
- How would the addition of two nurses to a clinic affect productivity?
- A payer recently added a pay-for-performance bonus for increasing the mammogram screening rate. How much additional revenue might an organization receive if it meets its goals?

The risk of taking only a performance reporting approach is that useful and unknown information in a large data warehouse may be missed. Data mining software uses three approaches to uncover this information: association, classification, and clustering.

Analysts use *association* algorithms in data mining to find interesting associations and correlations among large sets of data, where the presence of one set of items in a transaction implies the presence of others. Association is also called *market basket analysis*. Its most famous use was one convenience store chain's unexpected discovery of the strong correlation between diaper sales and beer sales on Fridays. Further analysis revealed that this phenomenon was due to "dad" being sent to the store to pick up diapers and deciding he might as well get some beer for the weekend. Retailers used this knowledge to position these goods in close proximity.

Classification defines groups within populations. Classification is useful in healthcare because most therapies are targeted to specific groups of patients (e.g., children under age 6 with asthma). Healthcare organizations already use many established grouping systems, such as DRGs, so the data mining classification tool is often used to develop non-standard groupings of similar patients. For example, patients with chronic disease could be classified according to their compliance with disease management protocols. Sophisticated marketing firms use data mining extensively to predict and shape buyer behavior; similar techniques will be used in the future to understand and shape patient compliance.

The final major tool for data mining is *cluster analysis*. Clustering differs from classification because it has no specific outcome or target variable but instead develops clusters of possibly related data items. Clustering is not yet used extensively in healthcare delivery. However, it is likely that in the future adventurous analysts will find unexpected and useful results by using cluster analysis on the large clinical databases now being created.

Although association, classification, and clustering are normally used on numeric data, modern data mining software also allows it to be used on text. This software removes common words (e.g., *it*, *the*, *and*) and then applies the data mining algorithms. *Text mining* can be used on stored documents and also on the web. *Web mining* identifies websites that may have content of interest and then scans the sites and applies the algorithms.

Benchmarking

In addition to evaluating internal data, organizations can benchmark to external organizations to gain useful insights and identify opportunities for improvement. Benchmarking can have two different purposes. The first is to compare organizational performance to similar organizations. Such comparison can help an organization identify areas of concern or areas where it possesses a competitive advantage.

A second purpose is to support improvement initiatives. In this case, the organization can benchmark against those considered best in class or known as the toughest competitors in a market. For example, Poudre Valley Health System, a 2008 Baldrige award winner, determined which hospitals were the national leaders in a number of clinical areas and then sent teams to benchmark their performance and translate this into improvements in its own system (National Institute of Standards and Technology 2009). The Baldrige award will be examined in more detail in Chapter 12.

In both purposes, benchmarking can be a major force in breaking down resistance to change in order to target areas for improvement and implement best practices.

Source of Benchmarks for Operational Data

Benchmarks can be obtained from many sources. Most professional associations maintain extensive data gathering and benchmarking programs. For example, the Medical Group Management Association provides one of the most complete physician practice benchmarking systems in the United States.

Commercial vendors also provide competitive benchmarking data at relatively affordable prices. For example, one vendor provides a pricing database that shows fee data by zip code for each current procedural terminology (CPT) code. The current fees for CPT codes in a geographic area are sorted and displayed at the 50th, 60th, 75th, 80th, 85th, 90th, and 95th percentiles (Ingenix 2009).

An advantage of using either professional association or commercial benchmarking databases is that these vendors have already identified key performance metrics to gather and report. However, a more strategic method to identify a limited set of key performance metrics is discussed in Chapter 5.

Examples of Operational Benchmarks

The following are some examples of operational and financial benchmarks for medical practices.

Practice Operations Metrics (Feltenberger and Gans 2008, p. 50)

- Staffing ratio: Total FTEs/Total FTE providers
- Medical support: Total FTE medical staff support/Total FTE physicians
- Average physician work relative value units (RVUs) per visit:

$$\frac{\text{(Sum of RVUs by all E and M codes + Sum of RVUs by all CPT codes)}}{\text{Total number of visits}}$$

Medical Practice Financial Metrics (Feltenberger and Gans 2008, p. 59)

- Net revenue per physician: Total net revenue/Total FTE physicians
- Medical revenue per physician:

$$\frac{\text{(Total medical revenue – Total operating costs)}}{\text{Total FTE physicians}}$$

Hospital Performance Metrics (Feltenberger and Gans 2008, p. 73)

- FTEs per adjusted occupied bed
- Case mix index
- Days in accounts receivable

Quality Measures and Benchmarks

In addition to operational and financial benchmarks, public reporting of quality results and related benchmarks is increasing dramatically.

The Centers for Medicare & Medicaid Services (CMS) publicly reports hospital performance at www.hospitalcompare.gov. It is also collecting physician data through the Physician Quality Reporting Initiative (PQRI). PQRI currently provides results and comparisons privately back to physicians and will publicly report participation in the program in 2010.

The other federal agency involved in quality improvement is the Agency for Healthcare Research and Quality (AHRQ), which sponsors numerous programs to develop and disseminate best practices and benchmarks. A new part of this effort is the Effective Health Care Program begun in 2009. Its goal is to produce effectiveness and comparative effectiveness research for clinicians, consumers, and policymakers. AHRQ is the lead federal agency charged with improving the quality, safety, efficiency, and effectiveness of healthcare for all Americans. Other organizations that are developing quality benchmarks and public reporting mechanisms include:

- The Leapfrog Group
- The Joint Commission
- National Quality Forum (NQF)
- National Committee for Quality Assurance (NCQA)

Analyzing Benchmarks

The use of benchmarks is both art and science, as organizations do not want to make significant changes based solely on benchmark data. Benchmark data should be one component of the environmental assessment in the strategic planning process described in Chapter 2.

When using benchmark data, the leadership challenge is to identify whom an organization should use as a comparison. Factors to consider are whether the benchmark data come from organizations with similar

- geography;
- patient demographics, ages, genders, and clinical risk profile;
- payer mix; and
- type of medical practice/specialty, hospital, and health plan.

When presenting benchmark data to an organization (and particularly to physicians), leadership must have a rock solid rationale for selecting a particular benchmark database.

Once a benchmark data set is selected, there are four standard methods of displaying the data:

- Absolute differences from the average (or median or deciles)
- Percentage difference from the average
- Median (used in large data sets)
- Mean plus measures of variability (e.g., standard deviation)

A more comprehensive method of displaying and analyzing these data is discussed in *Healthcare Operations Management*, Chapter 7.

NOTES FROM THE FIELD

HealthPartners—Performance Reporting

The BI function at HealthPartners is mature; the organization has a vice president for health informatics. Operational data from finance, claims, eligibility, EHRs, and other sources are loaded via ETL into a data warehouse where analysis is conducted using SAS. Some data are loaded monthly, while others are loaded daily. The primary use of the data warehouse is for performance reporting; 50 percent of the work of the BI unit supports operating departments.

Because HealthPartners is an integrated delivery system with its own large health plan, a number of its major BI projects have a broad scope. Examples include

- developing predictive analytics to identify patients for disease management,
- measuring and reporting population health, and
- providing targeted health plan data to employers.

Dean Health System—Benchmarking

Dean Health System has 60 healthcare facilities in southern and central Wisconsin. The system recently began a study of a large array of clinical utilization measures to identify waste in clinical processes. Leaders already had success cutting costs in administrative and operational processes with Lean-like process improvements, and they wanted to take a similar systematic approach to clinical expenditures.

Physicians were benchmarked on any clinical indicator for which an evidence-based guideline or external comparison was available, including admission rates for specific conditions, frequency of surgical intervention, length of stay for specific procedures, appropriateness of inpatient versus outpatient treatment, indications for imaging and lab testing, generic versus brand drug prescription, and many more.

On the prescription benchmark alone, physicians discovered significant areas with savings potential. For example, many prescriptions are routinely written for a 30-day supply, even when the patient needs the medication for a much longer time. For every 1 percent of prescriptions written for a 90-day supply rather than 30, $100,000 was saved in dispensing costs. This change improved patient service and reduced clinical utilization costs simultaneously. Altogether, Dean saved about $9 million in 2009, simply by discovering clinical inefficiencies that were not apparent to most providers. Dean's leadership reported that data alone were a major driver of changes in physician behavior.

Marshfield Clinic—Performance Reporting and Drill Down

The Marshfield Clinic has a highly developed data warehouse that allows it to generate reports such as that shown in Exhibit 3.14. This scatter chart shows all the patients with diabetes treated by one clinic in the Marshfield system and compares each patient's age to the number of diabetes measures not at goal. In addition, it allows drill-down detail to further investigate why some patients are outliers (this drill-down pop-up is shown in the exhibit).

Mayo Clinic—Data Mining

Mayo Clinic in Rochester, Minnesota, uses data mining to evaluate its operational procedures to target areas for improvement. In anticipation of bundled payments and penalties for readmissions within 30 days, Mayo Clinic leaders were interested in evaluating how many of their patients had a scheduled follow-up appointment. Mayo's EHR did not have a field for this information, so they turned to the discharge summary.

A data set consisting of discharge records was manually reviewed to determine whether the records contained follow-up appointment instructions. The same data set was evaluated for the same criteria using SAS Text Miner 3.1 software. The two assessments were compared to determine the accuracy of the text mining evaluation.

Exhibit 3.14
Marshfield Clinic
Scatter Chart
of Patient's Age
Versus Diabetes
Measures
Not at Goal

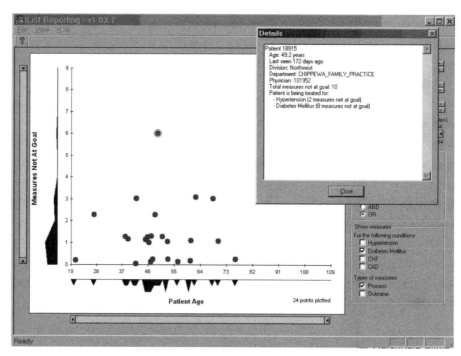

Source: Marshfield Clinic, Marshfield, WI. Used with permission.

Of the 6,481 discharge records reviewed, 3,576 (55.2 percent) were identified as containing all criteria for follow-up appointment instructions through manual review, 113 (3.2 percent) of which were missed through text mining. Text mining incorrectly identified 107 (3.7 percent) follow-up appointments that were not considered valid through manual review. In total, the text mining analysis concurred with the manual review in 96.6 percent of the appointment findings.

The Mayo researchers concluded that text mining of medical records can accurately detect whether elements of follow-up appointment instructions are documented in hospital discharge notes. The results also suggest that text mining software can be used to identify specific appointment criteria in a large number of textual medical records and thus save considerable resources required for manual abstraction in quality-related research and performance assessment.

The result of this research project provides a platform for Mayo to automatically track its clinic appointment follow-up after hospitalization, develop new strategies for improvement, and reduce its hospital readmission rate. Today, most automated EHRs contain a substantial amount of information stored as text. Mayo Clinic has shown that data mining can be a powerful tool for using text data for operations improvements.

VINCENT VALLEY HEALTHCARE

VVH planning staff knew that risk-based payments were going to increase in the future and that the VVH system had done well in the past with the original risk-based payment system, the DRG. However, they knew that these newer systems would require a higher level of understanding and precision.

Sameer Inampudi, director of business intelligence, began a project to expand VVH's data warehouse and upgrade its analytical capabilities. VVH had installed its EHR system two years previously and had worked through most of the implementation challenges. The data from this system were now being extracted and stored in a data warehouse. However, Inampudi and his staff understood that they needed to create a more comprehensive database. To that end, they began to add the following data elements to the main clinical warehouse:

- Financial billing and cost information related to each patient care episode
- Patient satisfaction data
- Human resources data related to staffing and workforce composition
- Budgeting data
- Data from other providers outside of VVH that provide care to VVH patients
- Benchmarking data, both quality and financial

Once these data were cleaned and loaded into the warehouse, some initial performance reporting could be done. The first analysis took advantage of the ETL process, which added episode of treatment groupings to each patient encounter as the data were loaded into the warehouse. Thereafter, a simple bar chart could be constructed for each ETG, showing average resources used per physician (see Exhibit 3.15).

The VVH staff also knew that patient compliance would make a large difference in these systems. Fortunately, the EHR was collecting data on mechanisms used to communicate with patients with chronic disease. VVH analysts used the data mining association tool to determine which methods seemed to best prompt patients to keep appointments. The tool looked at such data as appointment records, types of reminders sent, patient age, and patient zip code.

Exhibit 3.15
Average
Physician
Charges per
ETG—Chronic
Sinusitis with
Treatment,
Level 2 Severity

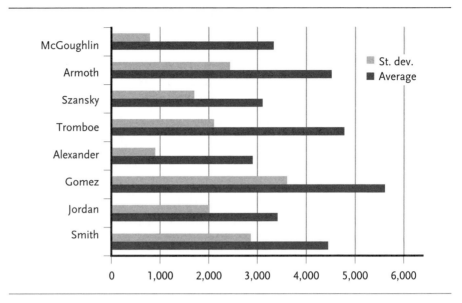

SUMMARY

To effectively develop a strategic plan, the planner must ensure that accurate data are an integral part of the process. The spread of information technology throughout healthcare organizations, particularly with the advent of the EHR, has greatly increased the amount of data available. The key is converting these data into information that is useful to strategy formulation.

Data are extracted from operational data systems and stored in data warehouses, which are designed to aid in the analysis of such data. Sophisticated performance reporting is now available, including graphics and predictive modeling. In addition, data mining can be used to find unexpected correlations and opportunities.

Also important is the comparison of internal performance with external benchmarks, especially the newly emerging clinical guidelines. Care must be taken when using benchmarks to ensure that truly similar organizations are included in the comparisons.

NOTES

1. The National Alliance for Health Information Technology has established the following definitions:
   - Electronic medical record (EMR): the electronic record of health-related information on an individual, that is created, gathered, managed, and consulted by licensed clinicians and staff from a single organization who are involved in the individual's health and care
   - Electronic health record (EHR): the aggregate electronic record of health-related information on an individual, that is created and gathered cumulatively across more than one healthcare organization and managed and consulted by licensed clinicians and staff involved in the individual's health and care
2. *Exegesis* is from the Greek "to lead out" and is a more detailed critical explanation or interpretation of text or fact.

CHAPTER 4

From Data Analysis to Focused Strategy

ALTHOUGH THE PROCESS of planning can be challenging, creating a data-based, flexible final plan is critical. In Chapter 2, alternative systems of strategic planning were reviewed. Chapter 3 detailed an approach to using business intelligence (BI) data analysis tools to identify strategic challenges and opportunities. This chapter outlines a methodology for integrating these two efforts to produce a strategic plan that can be effectively executed with the business tools outlined in Section II and the people and organizational skills detailed in Section III. Specifically, this chapter provides

- instruction on the use of scenario analysis to test the flexibility and robustness of the plan and
- an extensive example from VVH that integrates all the concepts from Section I (chapters 2, 3, and 4).

STATE OF THE ART

In Zuckerman's traditional model (see Exhibit 2.3), the strategic plan begins to take shape after internal and external reviews are completed (including appropriate internal data analysis and external benchmarking). This process consists of reviewing existing strategies, deleting strategies that are no longer relevant, and developing new strategies to meet challenges or opportunities. After a review of the consistency of these strategies with the organization's mission, they are translated into organizational and departmental goals.

"How do we get there?" is the next operational question. The business tools described in Section II provide a system for effective execution of these goals.

However, most strategic plans contain uncertainty about the future; scenario planning can improve the strategic plan and its subsequent execution.

SCENARIO PLANNING

As introduced in Chapter 2, scenario planning can improve an organization's strategic plan and test its robustness (i.e., its ability to respond effectively to unexpected internal or external environmental changes). The model described here is based on the work of Mats Lindgren and Hans Bandhold (2009).

The basic goals of scenario planning are to

- focus on minimizing the risks of maintaining "business as usual,"
- evaluate new business opportunities and paradigm shifts,
- support new business concepts and developments, and
- respond effectively to unexpected environmental changes.

Before beginning scenario planning, it is important to be clear on the organizational system that is being analyzed and the time horizons to be considered. The current situation should be well understood by the planning team through its analysis of internal and external data.

Tracking Trends

The first step in creating scenarios is to identify significant trends that will affect the organization during the plan's time horizon. A number of resources, such as Internet searches, professional associations and networks, focus groups, and expert panels, can be used to identify trends. Another useful source is *Futurescan* (American Hospital Association, Society for Healthcare Strategy and Market Development, American College of Healthcare Executives, and VHA 2010), which is published annually by Health Administration Press in collaboration with the Society for Healthcare Strategy and Market Development. The 2009 edition identified these trends as key drivers of strategy in the future:

- The globalization of healthcare
- The impact of an aging population
- The challenges and opportunities of the United States' foreign-born population
- Competition from new healthcare delivery vehicles
- The need to further engage physicians and more fully integrate them into leadership positions
- The growing role of employers in shaping the manner in which health insurance is provided and care is delivered

- The effect of transparency on patient safety and quality
- The impact of mandatory public reporting

Building Scenarios

Once trends have been identified, they should be ranked on two criteria: importance to the organization and uncertainty. The top two trends in uncertainty and importance then can be arrayed in a scenario cross (Exhibit 4.1). Although all the possible trends are ranked on uncertainty and importance, the scenario cross only displays the uncertainty axis. It is this range of uncertainties that is used to create the scenarios.

Four different scenarios emerge from these intersections. Good scenario planning practice suggests that each scenario should have a memorable title and a short descriptive paragraph.

As an example, consider two trends likely to be both important and uncertain in the future: payment reform and public reporting of quality. Payment reform is being demonstrated in a number of government programs and private health plans. Public reporting of quality and safety continues to expand, but it is currently being used only by professionals in the delivery system. However, as the general population becomes more facile with Internet tools, consumers may begin to use these resources to make decisions, which could affect market share. The scenario cross based on these trends is shown in Exhibit 4.2.

Scenario Descriptions

1. **Outcomes for dollars**—Payers unite and initiate substantial bonuses (10 to 20 percent) for achieving clinical outcomes. These payment systems are expanded beyond primary care to all specialties and are based partially on patient satisfaction. Only professionals routinely use public reporting websites; however, they use them to benchmark their own performance and identify best practices.
2. **Quality!**—Payers unite and initiate substantial bonuses (10 to 20 percent) for achieving clinical outcomes. These payment systems are expanded beyond primary care to all specialties and are based partially on patient satisfaction. Both patients and professionals now routinely use public reporting websites. The clinical outcomes of various providers are widely discussed on blogs and social networking websites. Many practices employ web marketing staff to correct errors and misstatements by patients.

**Exhibit 4.1
Scenario Cross**

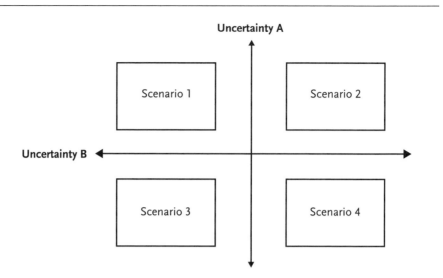

Source: Mats Lindgren and Hans Bandhold, *Scenario Planning*, revised edition, 2002, Palgrave Macmillan. Reproduced with permission of Palgrave Macmillen.

3. **Who cares?**—The system of quality reporting and payment changes very little. Only organizations that are strongly mission driven put extra resources into quality improvement. Finance departments continue to emphasize technical reimbursement strategies to maximize payments, such as installing systems to ensure the correct coding of bills.
4. **Marketers' paradise**—Although payment is not based on quality, many organizations are seeing significant shifts in market share that appear to be based on quality. The marketing and quality functions are merged in many healthcare delivery organizations. Boards of directors determine CEO compensation primarily on the basis of quality rankings.

Analysis

Once the scenarios have been created, each major strategy in an organization's plan can be evaluated against each scenario. Evaluation is based on the following criteria:

- **Effectiveness**—How well will this strategy work in this future scenario?
- **Competency**—How can the organization's talents be used to succeed in this scenario?
- **Complementarities**—Does this strategy support other strategies that will enable the organization to succeed in this scenario?

Exhibit 4.2
Scenario Cross
for Payment and
Public Reporting

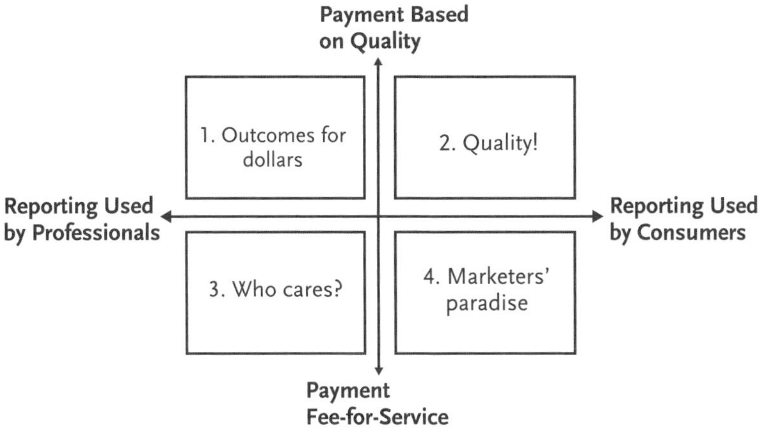

On the basis of this analysis, the strategic plan should be modified to respond as effectively as possible to each of the four scenarios. This final tune-up of the strategic plan will allow for agile responses to unanticipated shifts in the environment and robust application of the execution tools presented in sections II and III.

VINCENT VALLEY HEALTHCARE

After a series of meetings with top VVH staff and after reviewing internal and external data, Todd Stinson felt he could complete the VVH strategic plan. Although the plan was comprehensive, Stinson felt three strategies, if successful, would prompt sustained growth and success for VVH. The strategies he identified were development of a medical home, development of an accountable care organization (ACO), and implementation of bundled payments for inpatient care.

The Medical Home for Foothills Physicians

After a dinner meeting with Dr. Andresen, Dr. Moscone (chief medical officer of VVH) felt there were opportunities for collaboration with many of the primary care doctors in the Foothills area. A special interest of Dr. Andresen was the medical home concept, as she had been on the board of the state's Academy of Family Practice and had participated in some of the national committee work on the medical home. Fortunately, Stinson had negotiated a payment system for a medical home demonstration project with two of the major private payers and the state's Medicaid program and Children's Health Insurance Program. The VVH medical home would fit nicely into the federal ACO program once it became active.

The medical home is a concept, not a building. The general aim of the medical home is to continuously engage with the patient to ensure access, coordination of care, and shared decision making. This aim is achieved through changes to the organization and roles of the primary care clinic that enable seamless, coordinated, and efficient systems of care. Teamwork and effective use of health information technology are key components of these changes.

A recent study on the effectiveness of medical homes identified the importance of three key elements:

- Individualized and intense care for patients with chronic illness
- Efficient service provision
- Careful selection of specialists (based on quality and cost)

By carefully implanting these aspects of care, the medical homes studied reduced the total cost of care by 15 percent and improved quality. In addition, providers reported a "less frenetic clinical pace" (Milstein and Gilbertson 2009).

It was clear to Dr. Moscone that the Foothills physicians were not yet ready to make strong and binding ties to VVH but that VVH could be a reliable and cost-effective service partner. Many of these primary care doctors also saw the value in the medical home but did not have the capability to install health information technology or develop the teams needed for the medical home. Dr. Moscone felt that all of these tasks could be accomplished in a cost-effective manner—both for the individual practices and VVH.

The structure of the relationship between VVH and the Foothills' practices needed to be non-bureaucratic, with an emphasis on preserving physician autonomy. Therefore, Dr. Moscone decided to use a *learning style* planning system and recruited Jim Hanson to be the lead administrator for this initiative. The Foothills physicians would establish a steering committee that would meet monthly for dinner. Hanson would join the dinner to provide progress reports and recommend activities that could be part of implementing the medical home in these practices. One of Hanson's major tasks would be to work with each practice individually to solve problems or implement new features of the medical home. Once these activities gained enough commonality, they would be included in an informal strategic plan kept by Hanson and overseen by Dr. Moscone.

The goal for the coming year was to have ten practices join the network (approximately 25 physicians) and have medical home visits constitute 30 percent of the total patient care in each practice. The medical home strategy included the following initiatives:

1. Install a clinic-based EHR
2. Develop new processes for patient care within the medical home concept
3. Develop and test financial models of the medical home for each practice
4. Recruit new staff to be part of the medical home team (some staff shared among practices)
5. Train staff on use of the EHR
6. Train staff on new patient care processes that fit with the medical home model
7. Develop communication materials for patients
8. Update each practice's website

An ACO for VVH's Primary Care Network

Two private health plans approached Todd Stinson with the idea of developing an ACO to introduce a new product into the market. VVH would provide a tightly managed system of care, and customers could use this system for a relatively low cost or seek care outside the system for a higher copayment and deductible. The health plans proposed a contracting system to VVH that minimized the capitation risk but had a significant financial upside if the cost of healthcare delivered by VVH was lower than the community cost trend. Fortunately, the ACO structure that the health plans had in mind was similar to the federal ACO program, and both would reinforce a new emphasis on chronic disease management.

This initiative seemed to be a natural fit for VVH's own clinics, physicians, and medical center. The traditional Design and Planning schools were used to revise VVH's overall strategic plan and the ACO strategy initiative was added. Two goals for this initiative were determined: (1) Plan enrollment in the first year would exceed 10,000, and (2) the cost of care would be 2 percent lower than the community cost trend. Implementation of this strategy included the following major tasks:

1. Data mining and performance reporting to determine baseline performance of VVH
2. Benchmarking against the results of CMS's Physician Group Practice demonstration and Medicare health plans
3. Literature review and benchmarking of best practices in disease management

4. Development of new care processes and disease management approaches
5. Revisions to VVH's EHR to accommodate disease management
6. Recruitment of physicians to participate in care and disease management of ACO patients
7. Recruitment and selection of staff for the disease management function

Two uncertainties became apparent as these initiatives were reviewed. First, the performance of various disease management demonstration projects had been uneven (Linden and Adler-Milstein 2008), so the patient care and financial goals might be difficult to achieve. Second, VVH medical staff engagement and support were crucial to the success of this project, but there were many conflicting pressures on these physicians and it was unclear if they would have the ability and energy to focus on this new strategy. A scenario cross was constructed to explore these possibilities (Exhibit 4.3).

Scenarios

Staff do it all—Proven chronic disease management tools that are independent of the physicians are employed. Staff are careful to communicate effectively with physicians and update VVH's EHR in a disciplined manner. Staff leadership continues to test and improve methods of chronic disease management.

Increase market share—quickly!—With the full support of the medical staff and effective disease management tools, it appears that the VVH ACO will do well financially. This prospect provides a strong incentive to increase market share. A financial model is created to add benefits, such as dental and health club memberships for patients who receive over 80 percent of their care in the VVH ACO.

Minimal effort—Because the VVH disease management approaches do not appear to be particularly effective, the system strategy is to minimize overhead costs in the ACO until the target payment rates make ACO activities more attractive.

More research needed—Although the medical staff is actively engaged, the financial performance of the ACO is marginally successful. Therefore, a concerted effort is undertaken to review the literature and benchmark best practices from other leading healthcare systems.

Scenario 2 implies a rapid scale-up and implementation, while the other three scenarios suggest a more cautious approach. VVH felt it was important to first do the underlying research and benchmarking while determining

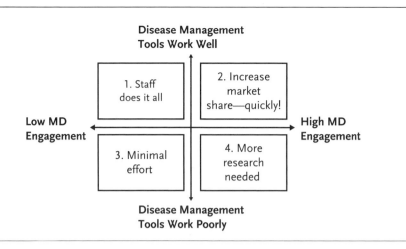

Exhibit 4.3
Scenario
Cross—
Physician
Engagement
Versus
Effectiveness
of Disease
Management

**Disease Management
Tools Work Well**

1. Staff
does it all

2. Increase
market
share—quickly!

**Low MD
Engagement**

**High MD
Engagement**

3. Minimal
effort

4. More
research
needed

**Disease Management
Tools Work Poorly**

medical staff commitment. Once these elements were determined to be positive, implementation of the ACO could begin.

Bundled Payments for VVH

VVH applied to CMS to participate in the Medicare Acute Care Episode (ACE) demonstration and was accepted. The ACE program pays a flat bundled rate for 9 orthopedic and 28 cardiac procedures. This fee includes hospital care, physician fees, and outpatient follow-up and rehabilitation. Twenty-two quality measures are reported each quarter to CMS. Physician payments can be increased by 25 percent if certain cost reduction targets and quality goals are met. Patients also receive a significant bonus, such as payments to offset premiums, to participate in this project (CMS 2010). After discussions with CMS staff, VVH staff were comfortable that the new bundled payment program in the healthcare reform law would be consistent with the ACE demonstration project.

The financial and marketplace opportunities for bundled payments moved VVH to include the ACE demonstration in its strategic plan. VVH had done well in analyzing DRGs[1] in its medical center and making changes in patient care pathways. However, the new bundled payment models required management of many resources outside the hospital walls—clinic visits, outpatient drugs, imaging, rehabilitation, and so on.

VVH set the following goals:

- Reduce readmissions within 30 days by 40 percent
- Increase quality measures for bundled payments by 20 percent
- Make or exceed cost targets by 5 percent on all bundled payments

This strategy would be led by Karen Bluhm, VVH's chief nursing officer. To meet these goals, VVH would have to complete the following major tasks:

1. Determine membership and initiate a project team for this strategy
2. Acquire external provider data and integrate them into the VVH data warehouse
3. Do performance reporting and data mining on the appropriate DRGs and related bundled payment groups
4. Use medical staff, benchmarking, literature reviews, and other sources to identify opportunities for improvement
5. Solicit cooperation and new relationships with clinicians outside of the VVH system who are providing care for VVH-admitted patients
6. Revise the EHR to include clinical decision support modules as part of each bundled payment group and targeted DRG
7. Develop an outreach office to coordinate care after discharge
8. Implement and monitor results, and make changes as needed

SUMMARY

As discussed in chapters 2 and 3, a number of approaches can be used to create strategic plans. Those most commonly used in healthcare include the Design, Planning, and Learning schools. To effectively develop these plans, internal data analysis through the use of data warehouses should be employed and external benchmarks evaluated.

Once an initial strategy is determined, scenario analysis can be used to evaluate its robustness. First, major trends are identified, and two are selected to form a scenario cross (high versus low probability of occurrence). A scenario is created and named for each of the quadrants. Each strategy is tested against each of the scenarios to determine its effectiveness, the organization's ability to implement it, and how it complements other strategies. If the proposed strategy is not robust with regard to these alternative scenarios, it is adjusted.

NOTE

1. Medicare classifies patient cases into one of approximately 500 Diagnosis Related Groups (DRGs). Medicare bases its reimbursement on the DRG to which a patient case is assigned. This payment is fixed but may be adjusted for the severity of the admission.

SECTION II

TOOLS

We become what we behold. We shape our tools and then our tools shape us.

Marshall McLuhan, Canadian educator, scholar, philosopher

CHAPTER 5

The Balanced Scorecard

As shown in Section I, most healthcare organizations can develop good strategic plans, but they frequently fail to implement them.

This chapter demonstrates how to resolve this problem by using the balanced scorecard to consistently move strategy to action. First, traditional management systems are examined and their failures explored. Next, the theory of the balanced scorecard is reviewed and its application to healthcare organizations explained. Finally, practical steps to implement and maintain a balanced scorecard system are provided.

This chapter covers

- problems in today's management systems,
- using a balanced scorecard to move strategy to action,
- monitoring strategy from the four perspectives,
- identifying key initiatives to achieve a strategic objective,
- developing a strategy map that links initiatives,
- identifying and measuring leading and lagging indicators for each initiative,
- the balanced scorecard as a management system, and
- common implementation issues.

STATE OF THE ART

Why Do Today's Management Tools Fail?

Historically, most organizations have been managed with three primary tools: strategic plans, financial reports, and operational reports. In this traditional system, the first step is to create a strategic plan, which is usually updated annually. Next, a budget and an operational plan are created. The operational plan is sometimes referred to as the tactical plan; it provides more detailed task descriptions with timelines and expected outcomes. Senior management monitors the organization's performance through the financial and operational reports. If managers encounter deviations from expected performance, they take corrective action.

Although theoretically easy to grasp, this management system frequently fails for a number of common reasons. Organizations are awash in operating data, and they make no effort to identify key metrics. The strategic plans, financial reports, and operational reports are all created by different departments, and each report is reviewed in different time frames, often by different managers. Finally, the reports do not connect with one another.

These issues are some of the root causes of poor execution. If strategies are not linked to "actionable" items, operations will not change, nor will the financial results. In addition, strategic plans are frequently not linked to departmental or individual goals and reside only on the shelf in the executive suite.

Frequently, the time frame of strategy execution is also problematic. Financial reports tend to be timely and accurate but reflect only the current reporting period. Unfortunately, reviews of these reports do not encourage the long-term strategic allocation of resources (e.g., a major capital expenditure) that may require multiple-year investments. A good financial outcome in the current month is probably due to an action that occurred many months in the past. The cumulative result of these problems is poor execution, which leads to poor outcomes.

Robert Kaplan and David Norton

In the early 1990s, Robert Kaplan and David Norton (1996) undertook a study to examine how companies measure their performance. The growing sophistication of companywide information systems was beginning to provide senior management with executive information systems that featured elaborate displays and "dashboards" of company performance. The original purpose of Kaplan and Norton's study was to understand and document this trend.

However, their study uncovered several reporting practices that many leading companies were using to measure their performance. These firms looked at their operations from a number of perspectives that, together, provided a "balanced scorecard." The essential elements of this work were first reported in *The Balanced Scorecard: Translating Strategy into Action* (Kaplan and Norton 1996) and *The Strategy-Focused Organization* (Kaplan and Norton 2001). They have continued to publish books and articles to broaden the understanding and application of this technology.

The key element of the balanced scorecard is, of course, balance. An organization can be viewed from many perspectives, but Kaplan and Norton identified four common perspectives from which an organization must examine its operations (Exhibit 5.1):

1. Financial
2. Customer
3. Internal process and innovation
4. Employee learning and growth

An organization is viewed from each perspective, so different measures of performance are important. Every perspective in a complete balanced scorecard contains a set of objectives, measures, targets, and actions. Each measure in each perspective must be linked to the organization's overall strategy. The indicators of performance in each of the four perspectives must be both leading (predicting the future) and lagging (reporting on past performance). Indicators also must be obtained from inside the organization and from the external environment.

Although many think of the balanced scorecard as a reporting technique, its true power comes from its ability to link strategy to action. Balanced scorecard practitioners develop strategy maps that link projects and actions to outcomes. These maps display the "theory of the company" and can be evaluated and fine-tuned with many of the quantitative techniques described in *Healthcare Operations Management*.

Elements of the Balanced Scorecard System

A complete balanced scorecard system has the following elements, explained in detail in the following sections:

- Organizational mission, vision, and strategy
- Perspectives
  - ~ Financial
  - ~ Customer
  - ~ Internal business process
  - ~ Learning and growing

Exhibit 5.1
The Four
Perspectives in
the Balanced
Scorecard

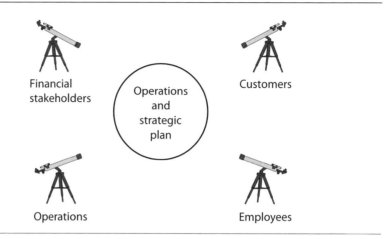

Financial
stakeholders

Operations
and
strategic
plan

Customers

Operations

Employees

- Strategy maps
- Themes
- Strategic alignment—top to bottom
- Processes for identifying targets, resources, initiatives, and budgets
- Balanced scorecard management system
- Feedback and the strategic learning process

Strategy Development

The balanced scorecard system presupposes that an organization has an effective mission, vision, and strategy in place. Section I of this book provided a number of approaches to developing an effective strategy. However, it is important that each strategy be clearly defined and have quantitative goals no matter which planning approach was used to create it.

For example, a traditional Design and Planning School strategy might be to increase revenue by 6 percent through the growth of retail and consumer-directed services. This strategy was identified after a careful review of retail and marketing data available in the organization's data warehouse.

A Learning School strategy might be based on the unanticipated opportunity to acquire a practice of five physicians. The goal for this new strategy would be a revenue increase of 3.5 percent for the organization with no reduction in operating margin. In both schools, the strategy is specific and includes measurable outcomes.

With an effective strategic plan in place, the next step is to begin evaluating its implementation as viewed from each of the four perspectives (financial, customer, operational, and learning and growing). Placing a perspective at the top of a balanced scorecard strategy map means that results in this perspective contain the final outcomes desired by the organization. In most organizations, the financial view is the top perspective. Therefore, the initiatives undertaken in the other three perspectives should result in positive financial performance.

The Four Perspectives

Financial Perspective
Although the other three perspectives and their associated areas of activity should lead to outstanding financial performance, the financial perspective also includes some specific initiatives. The major focuses for financial initiatives and financial measurement include

- revenue growth,
- cost reduction and/or productivity increases,
- asset utilization and investment strategy improvements, and
- risk reduction through diversity (revenue sources, cost drivers, and assets).

If an organization is in a growth mode, the focus should be on increasing revenue to accommodate growth. If it is operating in a relatively stable environment, the organization may choose to emphasize profitability. If the organization is stable and profitable, the focus can shift to investment—in both physical assets and human capital. Another major strategy in the financial domain is the diversification of revenues and expenditures to minimize financial risk.

Customer Perspective and Market Segmentation
The second perspective is to view an organization's operations from the customer's point of view. In most healthcare operations, the customer is the patient. Integrated health organizations, however, may operate health plans; their customers are then employers or the government. Many hospitals and clinics also consider their community, in total, as the customer. The physician could also be seen as the customer in many hospital organizations.

Once the customers are identified, it is helpful to segment them into smaller groups and determine the "value" proposition that will be delivered to each customer segment. Example market segments are patients with chronic illnesses (e.g., diabetes, congestive heart failure), obstetric care, sports medicine, cancer care, emergency care, Medicaid patients, small employers, and referring primary care physicians.

Once market segments have been determined, a number of traditional measures of marketplace performance may be applied, the most prominent being market share. Customers should be individually tracked and measured in terms of retention and acquisition; it is always easier to retain an existing customer than to attract a new one. Customer satisfaction and profitability are also useful measures.

Internal Business Process Perspective

The third perspective in the balanced scorecard is that of internal business processes, or operations. The internal business process perspective has three major components: innovation, ongoing process improvement, and post-sale service.

A well-functioning healthcare organization has a purposeful innovation process. The first step in an organized innovation process is to identify a potential market segment. Then, two primary questions need to be answered:

- What benefits will customers value in tomorrow's market?
- How can the organization innovate to deliver these benefits?

Once these questions have been researched and answered, product creation can commence.

Standard innovation measures used in many industries outside healthcare include percentage of sales from new products, percentage of sales from proprietary products, new product introductions per year, time to develop new products, and time to break even.

The case for process improvement and operations excellence is now well understood in most progressive healthcare organizations. *Healthcare Operations Management* provides a thorough review of contemporary tools for process improvement, including Lean Six Sigma and process simulation with computer-aided discrete event simulation.

The final aspect of the operations perspective is post-sales, an area poorly executed in most healthcare delivery organizations. Good post-service systems provide patients with follow-up information on the service they received. For example, patients with chronic diseases should be contacted periodically with reminders about diet, medication use, and the need to schedule follow-up visits. An outstanding post-sale system also finds opportunities for improvement in the service and possible innovations for the future.

Learning and Growing Perspective

The final perspective from which to view an organization is that of learning and growing. To effectively execute a strategy, employees must be motivated and have the necessary tools to succeed. Therefore, successful organizations make substantial investments in this aspect of their operations. Chapters 9 and 10 review a number of approaches to improving organizational culture and employee engagement.

Linking Balanced Scorecard Measures to Strategy

Once expected objectives and their related measures are determined for each perspective, initiatives to meet these goals must be developed. An initiative can be a simple action or a large project. Chapters 6, 7, and 9 provide a comprehensive approach to effective initiative execution. It is important to logically link each initiative to the desired outcome through a series of cause-and-effect statements, which are usually "if-then" constructions. For example:

- *If* the wait time in the emergency department is decreased, *then* the patient will be more satisfied.
- *If* an admitting process is improved through the use of automation, *then* the final collection rate will improve.
- *If* an optically scanned wristband is used in conjunction with an electronic health record, *then* medication errors will decline.

Each initiative should have measures associated with it, and every measure selected for a balanced scorecard should be an element in a chain of cause-and-effect relationships that communicate the organization's strategy.

Outcomes and Performance Drivers

Selecting appropriate measures for each initiative is critical. There are two basic types of indicators. Outcome indicators, familiar to most managers, are also termed "lagging indicators" because they result from earlier actions. Outcome indicators tend to be generic instead of tightly focused. Healthcare operations examples include profitability, market share, and patient satisfaction. The other type of indicator is a performance driver, or "leading indicator." These indicators predict the future and are specific to an initiative and the organization's strategy. For example, a performance driver measure could be waiting time in the emergency department. A drop in waiting time should predict an improvement in the outcome indicator, patient satisfaction.

Strategy Maps

As discussed, a set of initiatives should be linked together by if-then statements to achieve a desired outcome. Both outcome and performance driver indicators should be determined for each initiative. They can be displayed graphically in a strategy map, which may be organized into the four perspectives, with learning and growing at the bottom and financial at the top. A general strategy map for any organization includes these statements:

- *If* employees have skills, tools, and motivation, *then* they will improve operations.
- *If* operations are improved and marketing is also improved, *then* customers will buy more products and services.
- *If* customers buy more products and services and operations are run efficiently, *then* the organization's financial performance will improve.

Exhibit 5.2 shows a strategy map indicating these general initiatives.

The strategy map is enhanced if each initiative also contains the strategic objective, measure used, and target results that the organization hopes to achieve. Each causal pathway from initiative to initiative needs to be clear and quantitative if possible. A simple strategy map of patient flow in the emergency department is shown in Exhibit 5.3.

The first required steps in this strategy are forming a project team (chapters 6 and 7) and learning how to use Lean Six Sigma process improvement tools. Then, the team can begin analyzing patient flow and implementing changes to improve flow. Once these changes are implemented, waiting time for 90 percent of patients should not exceed 30 minutes. Reduced waiting time should contribute to greater patient satisfaction, which then should lead to growth in market share and increased net revenue. Here are the more formal cause-and-effect statements:

- *If* emergency department staff undertake educational activities to learn project management and Lean Six Sigma, *then* they can effectively execute a patient flow improvement project.
- *If* a patient flow project is undertaken and non–value added time is reduced by 30 percent, *then* the waiting time for most patients should never exceed 30 minutes.
- *If* the waiting time for most patients never exceeds 30 minutes, *then* they will be highly satisfied, and high patient satisfaction will drive more patients to the hospital and boost its market share.

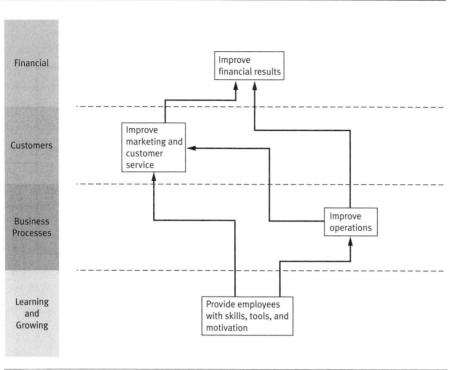

**Exhibit 5.2
General Strategy
Map**

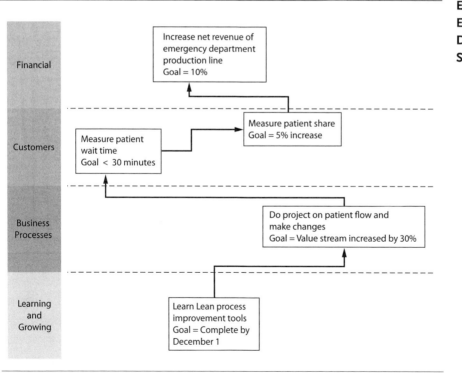

**Exhibit 5.3
Emergency
Department
Strategy Map**

- *If* the emergency department market share increases, *then* net revenue will increase.

Themes and Synergy

Implementation of the various initiatives in the strategy map often overlap a number of departments. One way to clarify accountability is to group each initiative into a larger theme, such as "achieve operational excellence" or "build brand and grow market share." When these themes are identified, one senior individual can be assigned accountability for a set of initiatives on a strategy map. That person can also become each initiative's project sponsor.

Synergy among many operating units can also be achieved through coordination and shared services. The electronic health record is a shared service and most likely a strategic initiative on most healthcare organizations' strategy maps. This initiative can be the key to developing organization synergies and operational efficiencies.

Modifications by Healthcare Organizations

The balanced scorecard has been modified by many healthcare organizations, most commonly by placing the customer or patient at the top of the strategy map. Finance then becomes a means to achieve superior patient outcomes and satisfaction. Some organizations add perspectives such as "community" or "research and teaching."

Cascading Strategy Maps and Scorecards

The balanced scorecard can be used at many different levels in an organization. However, departmental scorecards should link to the divisional, and ultimately the corporate, level. Each scorecard should be linked upward and downward. For example, an obstetric initiative to increase revenue from normal childbirth should be linked to the corporate-level objective of overall increased revenue. Although strategy maps are optional at the department level, scorecards should be carefully crafted and monitored at all operating levels to achieve effective execution.

Sometimes it is difficult to specifically link a departmental strategy map to corporate objectives. In this case, the department head must make a more general linkage by stating how a departmental initiative will influence a particular corporate goal. For example, improving the quality of the hospital laboratory testing system will generally influence the corporate objective that patients should perceive that the hospital provides the highest level of quality care.

The development and operation of scorecards at each level of an organization require disciplined communication and can provide an incentive for individuals to take action. Balanced scorecards can also be used to communicate with an organization's external stakeholders. A well-implemented balanced scorecard system will be integrated with individual employee goals and the organization's performance management system.

Targets, Resources, Initiatives, and Budgets

A balanced scorecard strategy map consists of a series of linked initiatives. Each initiative should have a quantitative measure, a target budget, and resource allocations (e.g., employees assigned to the initiative). Initiatives can reside in one department, but they are frequently cross-departmental. Many initiatives are projects; in such cases, the process for successful project management (chapters 6 and 7) should be followed. A well-implemented balanced scorecard will also link carefully to an organization's budget, particularly if initiatives and projects are expected to consume considerable operating or capital resources.

The use of the balanced scorecard does not obviate the use of additional operating statistics. Many other operating and financial measures still need to be collected and analyzed. If the performance of any of these measures deviates substantially from its expected target, a new strategy and initiative may be needed. The data warehousing and performance reporting tools explained in Chapter 3 should be used for this purpose.

Displaying Results

The actual scorecard tracks and communicates the results of each initiative. (Chapter 3 provides examples of many types of visual display.) A challenge for most organizations is to collect the data to display in the scorecard. Because the scorecard should have fewer than 20 measures, a simple solution is to assign data collection and display responsibility to one individual. This person develops efficient methods to collect the data and determines effective methods to display them.

A Strategy Management System—Ensuring That the Balanced Scorecard Works

Once a balanced scorecard system is created it must be monitored closely. Kaplan and Norton (2008) recommend that management teams divide their routine meetings into three types: operational reviews, strategy reviews, and strategy testing/adaptation. The operational meeting is held frequently (e.g., weekly) and is designed to respond to short-term problems and promote improvements. The strategy review meeting is held monthly and focuses on monitoring and fine-tuning the existing strategy map. The strategy testing/adaptation meeting should be held at least annually and more frequently if the environment is changing rapidly. These meetings are designed to improve or transform the existing strategy, develop new initiatives and revised maps, and authorize needed expenditures.

The explicit purpose of the balanced scorecard is to ensure the successful execution of an organization's strategy. But what if it does not achieve the desired results? There are two possible causes.

The first, most obvious, problem is that an initiative is simply not achieving its targeted results. For example, the emergency department's patient flow project may not be able to decrease non–value added time by 30 percent. In that case, the hospital may have to add another initiative, such as engaging a consultant. This measure will need to be carefully monitored and frequently posted on the scorecard.

The second, more complex, problem occurs when the successful execution of an initiative does not lead to achievement of the next linked target. For example, although waiting times in the emergency department are decreased, the emergency department may not gain market share. The solution to this problem is to reconsider the cause-and-effect relationships.

An organization should review its results and strategy map at least quarterly and revise its strategy annually, usually as part of the budgeting process.

Implementation Issues

Two common challenges occur when implementing balanced scorecards: (1) determination and development of metrics and (2) initiative prioritization.

The balanced scorecard is a quantitative tool and, therefore, requires data systems that generate timely information. Each initiative on a strategy map should have quantitative measures, and there should be an even mix of leading and lagging measures.

Each initiative should have a target as well. However, setting targets is an art: Too timid a goal will not move an organization forward, and too aggressive a goal will discourage its staff.

A number of sources should be used to construct targets. Sources include internal company operating data, executive interviews, internal and external strategic assessments, customer research, industry averages, and benchmarking data. Targets can be incremental (e.g., increase productivity in a nursing unit by 10 percent in the next 12 months), or they can be "stretch goals," which are possible but require extraordinary effort to achieve (e.g., improve compliance with evidence-based guidelines for 98 percent of diabetes patients). A scorecard with too many measures and initiatives is confusing; even the most sophisticated organizations therefore limit their measures to 20 or fewer.

The second major implementation challenge is the prioritization of initiatives. Most organizations do not lack for current initiatives or projects, and influential leaders in the organization often propose many more. Niven (2002) suggests a methodology to manage this phenomenon:

1. Inventory all current initiatives taking place in the organization
2. Map those initiatives to the objectives of the balanced scorecard
3. Consider eliminating non-strategic initiatives, and develop missing initiatives
4. Prioritize the remaining initiatives

Most organizations will never be able to perfectly align their balanced scorecard goals with all of their initiatives. However, the closer the alignment, the more likely the organization is to achieve its strategic objectives.

NOTES FROM THE FIELD

SMDC Strategy Map and Balanced Scorecard

SMDC Health System (St. Mary's Hospital/Duluth Clinic) is one of the most sophisticated users of the balanced scorecard in healthcare; the health system has been inducted into the Balanced Scorecard Hall of Fame. Exhibit 5.4 is the strategy map for SMDC. Note the four themes of service excellence, clinical excellence, operational excellence, and innovation/growth.

The actual scorecard at SMDC is sophisticated and allows all goals to be tracked dynamically. The initiative P4 articulates the goal: "We will deliver safe, coordinated care through teams that include the patient to achieve best

Exhibit 5.4 SMDC Strategy Map

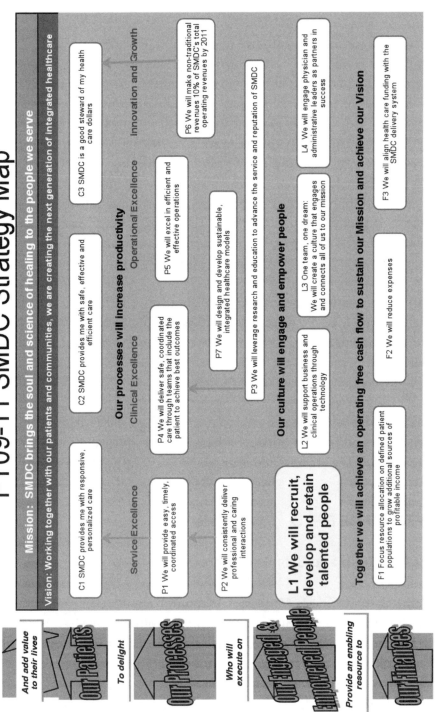

FY09-11 SMDC Strategy Map

Mission: SMDC brings the soul and science of healing to the people we serve

Vision: Working together with our patients and communities, we are creating the next generation of integrated healthcare

Our processes will increase productivity

Clinical Excellence   Operational Excellence   Innovation and Growth

Service Excellence

C1 SMDC provides me with responsive, personalized care

C2 SMDC provides me with safe, effective and efficient care

C3 SMDC is a good steward of my health care dollars

P6 We will make non-traditional revenues 10% of SMDC's total operating revenues by 2011

P1 We will provide easy, timely, coordinated access

P4 We will deliver safe, coordinated care through teams that include the patient to achieve best outcomes

P5 We will excel in efficient and effective operations

L4 We will engage physician and administrative leaders as partners in success

P2 We will consistently deliver professional and caring interactions

P7 We will design and develop sustainable, integrated healthcare models

Our culture will engage and empower people

P3 We will leverage research and education to advance the service and reputation of SMDC

L1 We will recruit, develop and retain talented people

L2 We will support business and clinical operations through technology

L3 One team, one dream: We will create a culture that engages and connects all of us to our mission

Together we will achieve an operating free cash flow to sustain our Mission and achieve our Vision

F1 Focus resource allocation on defined patient populations to grow additional sources of profitable income

F2 We will reduce expenses

F3 We will align health care funding with the SMDC delivery system

And add value to their lives
Our Patients

To delight
Our Processes

Who will execute on
Our Engaged & Empowered People

Provide an enabling resource to
Our Finances

Copyright © 2009 by St. Mary's/Duluth Clinic Health System, Duluth, MN. Used with permission.

**Exhibit 5.5
Drill-Down
Reporting of
Individual
Physician
Performance
at SMDC**

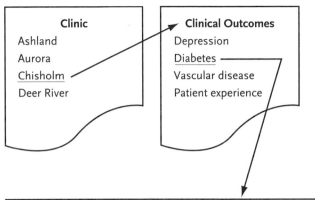

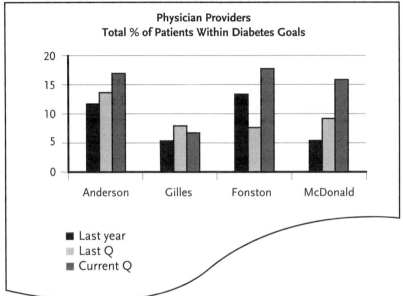

Physician Providers
Total % of Patients Within Diabetes Goals

(1) Maintain blood pressure less than 130/80; (2) lower LDL or "bad" cholesterol to less than 100 mg/dL; (3) control blood sugar so that A1c level is less than 7%; (4) don't smoke; (5) take an aspirin daily, for those ages 40 and older.

outcomes." Performance is tracked down to the individual physician level through the use of drill-down scorecards (see Exhibit 5.5).

VINCENT VALLEY HEALTHCARE

Jim Hanson decided that a strategy map would be useful as he began working with the Foothills physicians on developing the medical home capability. The map helped communicate the strategy and specify the metrics for success (Exhibit 5.6).

Exhibit 5.6 Tasker Foothills Medical Home Strategy Map

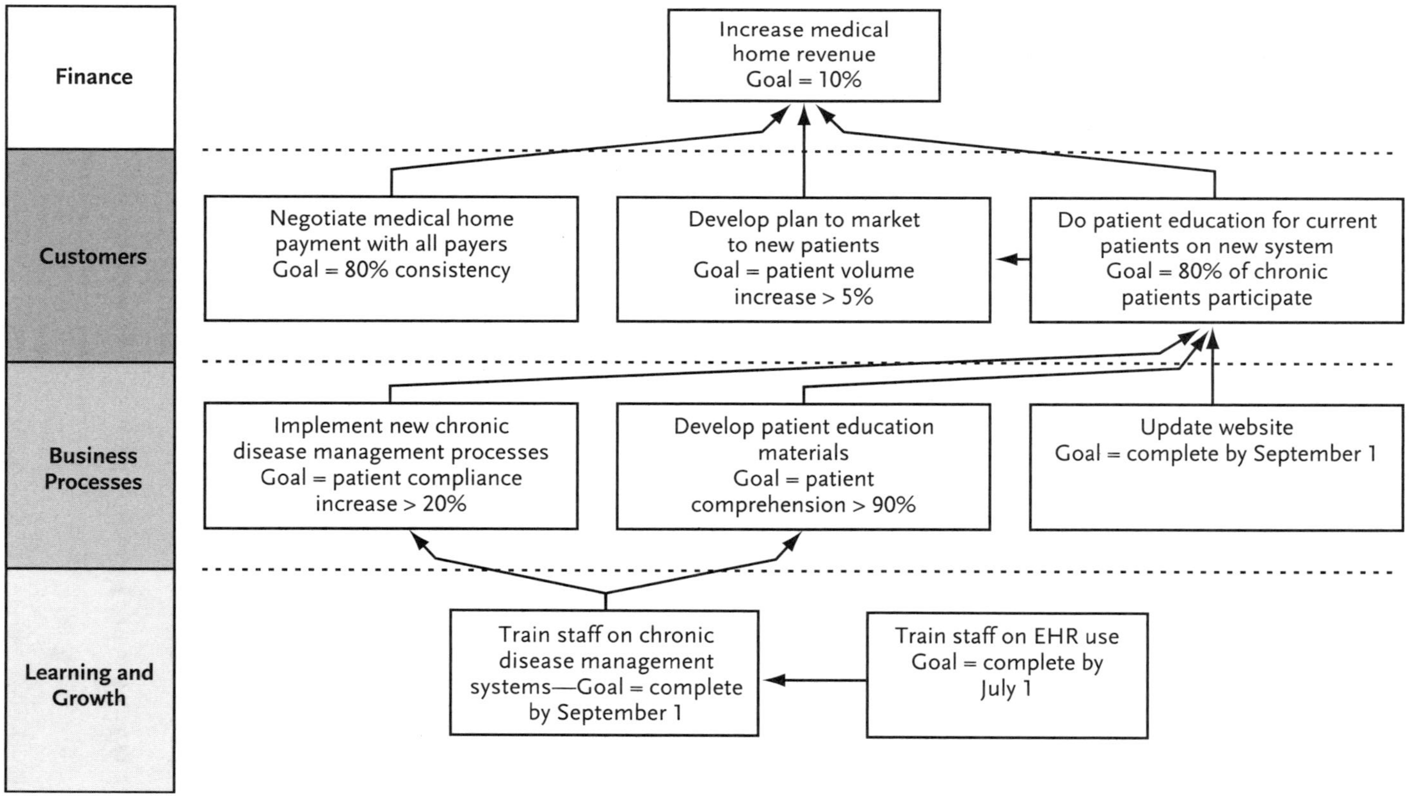

Finance	
Customers	
Business Processes	
Learning and Growth	

Increase medical home revenue
Goal = 10%

Negotiate medical home payment with all payers
Goal = 80% consistency

Develop plan to market to new patients
Goal = patient volume increase > 5%

Do patient education for current patients on new system
Goal = 80% of chronic patients participate

Implement new chronic disease management processes
Goal = patient compliance increase > 20%

Develop patient education materials
Goal = patient comprehension > 90%

Update website
Goal = complete by September 1

Train staff on chronic disease management systems—Goal = complete by September 1

Train staff on EHR use
Goal = complete by July 1

RESOURCES

The companion website to this book, ache.org/books/execution, contains a downloadable strategy map and linked scorecard. It also has a number of videos that demonstrate how to use and modify these tools.

SUMMARY

Most organizations have difficulty implementing their strategic plans due to the disconnect between strategy, operations, and outcomes (financial, operational, sales, and so on). Used together, a balanced scorecard and accompanying strategy maps are an integrated strategy management system that helps organizations overcome this challenge.

The first step in using this tool is to view the organization's strategy from four perspectives: financial, customer/patient, operations, and workforce. In each of these viewpoints, the organization can identify initiatives that will help it achieve its strategic goals. The metrics and targets set for each initiative become the actual scorecard. The second step is to link the initiatives together to create a strategy map that shows the logic of the connections and the interdependence among them.

The scorecard's results should be monitored frequently to ensure that initiatives are effectively implemented. The effectiveness of the strategy map is reviewed at least annually to ensure that the logic of the strategy map is delivering expected results.

CHAPTER 6

Project Management

WHETHER WE ARE painting a bedroom at home or adding a 150-bed wing to a hospital, effective project execution depends on effective project management. This chapter outlines the science of project management and its formal application as defined by the Project Management Institute.

Chapter 7 provides an overview of variations and modifications to this formal method. However, for complex, large, or high-risk projects, this formal methodology should be followed. The major topics covered in this chapter include

- selecting and chartering projects;
- using stakeholder analysis to set project requirements;
- developing a work breakdown structure (WBS) and schedule;
- using Microsoft Project to develop project plans and monitor their implementation;
- managing project communications, change control, and risk;
- selecting the project team; and
- establishing a project management office.

This chapter is organized somewhat differently from other chapters in this book in that the Vincent Valley Healthcare System is used throughout to illustrate the details of the project management process.

Once an organization's strategy has been determined and converted into strategy maps, it often becomes evident that some initiatives on the map are actually large projects. An ability to successfully move this type of a project forward while meeting time and budget goals is a distinguishing characteristic of the high-quality, highly competitive healthcare organization.

Effective project management enables healthcare organizations to quickly develop new clinical services, fix major operating problems, reduce expenses, and provide new consumer-directed products to their patients.

The problems with poor project management became apparent in the defense industry after World War II. Many new weapons systems were wildly over budget and late and did not perform as expected. The automated baggage conveyor system at Denver International Airport is another frequently cited example of a poorly managed project. In 2005, after ten years of malfunctions and high maintenance costs, the airport stopped using it. Baggage is now handled manually.

A response to this problem was the gradual development of project management as a discipline, culminating in the establishment of the Project Management Institute (PMI) in 1969 (www.PMI.org). The 1950s can be characterized as the beginning of the modern project management era; new mathematical and scheduling techniques were first used by the Defense Department for the Polaris nuclear missile submarine project. Today, PMI has more than 110,000 members, and more than 50,000 of them are certified as Project Management Professionals (PMPs).

PMI members have developed the Project Management Body of Knowledge (PMBOK) (Project Management Institute 2008), which details best practices for successful project management. Much as evidence-based medicine delineates the most effective treatment of specific clinical conditions, the PMBOK provides science-based, field-tested guidelines.[1] This chapter is based on PMBOK principles (fourth edition) as applied to healthcare. Healthcare professionals who spend much of their time leading projects should consider using resources available through PMI; for some, PMP certification may be appropriate.

DEFINITION OF A PROJECT

A project is a onetime set of activities that culminates in a desired outcome. Therefore, activities that occur repeatedly, such as making appointments for patients in a clinic, are not projects. However, the installation of new software to upgrade this capability would be a project. A major process improvement effort to reduce phone hold time would also qualify as a project.

Once an issue or initiative has been identified as a project, a number of approaches can be used. For example, a simple operating problem (e.g., a software upgrade for all computers in a clinic) can be assigned to a manager; it then becomes part of his workflow. However, projects that are complex and have high organizational value need the discipline of formal project management. Many of the strategic initiatives on an organization's balanced scorecard should use project management methodology.

A well-managed project includes a specified scope of work, expected outcomes and performance levels, a budget, and a detailed work breakdown tied to a schedule. It also includes a formal change procedure, communications plan, and risk management plan. Finally, all good projects include a conclusion process and a plan for redeployment of staff.

Many high performing organizations also have a formal executive-level chartering process for projects and a project management office to monitor enterprise-wide project activities. The project management office is outlined in the last section of this chapter. Some healthcare organizations (e.g., health plans) have a substantial share of their operating resources invested in projects at any one time.

For effective execution of a project, PMI recommends three elements be present. A *project charter* begins the project and addresses stakeholder needs. A *project scope statement* identifies project outcomes, timelines, and budget in detail. Finally, a *project plan* includes scope management, work breakdown, schedule management, cost management, quality control, staffing management, communications, risk management, procurement, and the closeout process. Exhibit 6.1 displays the relationships between these elements.

PROJECT SELECTION AND CHARTERING

Project Selection

Most organizations have many projects vying for attention, funding, and senior executive support. The annual budget and strategic planning process serves as a useful vehicle for prioritizing projects in many organizations. The balanced scorecard (Chapter 5) helps leaders identify worthwhile strategic projects. External forces (e.g., new Medicare rules) or clinical innovations (e.g., new imaging technologies), however, usually conspire to present an organization's leaders with a list of projects too long for successful implementation. Niven (2005) provides a useful tool for prioritizing projects (Exhibit 6.2).

To use this tool, a senior planning group scores each potential project on the basis of the following criteria:

- Fit with the organization's strategy
- Financial benefit and cost
- Need for key personnel

**Exhibit 6.1
Complete Project
Management
Process**

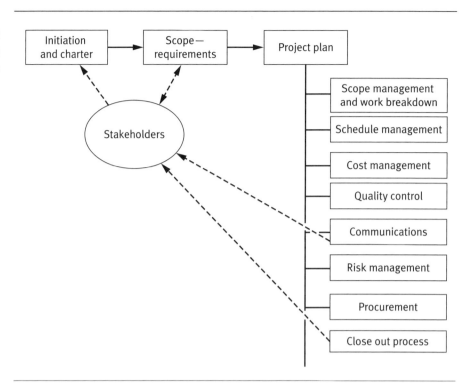

- Time required
- Positive effect on other projects

A scale of one (low) to ten (high) is typically used. Each criterion is also weighted; the scores are multiplied by their weight for each criterion and summed over all of the criteria. In Exhibit 6.2, Project A has a higher total score due to its importance to the organization's strategy. Such a ranking methodology prevents organizations from committing resources to projects that may have a powerful internal champion but do not advance the organization's overall strategy. This matrix can be modified with other categories and weights on the basis of an organization's current needs.

With the rise of comparative effectiveness research and the public reporting of quality, a large number of clinical project opportunities will easily be identified. Chapter 7 explores the challenge of prioritizing and implementing these projects in more depth.

Project Charter

Once a project is identified for implementation, it needs to be chartered. Four factors interact to constrain the execution of a project charter: time,

Exhibit 6.2
Project
Prioritization
Matrix

Criteria	Weight	Project A points	Project A score	Project B points	Project B score
Linkage to strategy	45%	7	3.15	1	0.45
Financial gain	15%	5	0.75	10	1.5
Project cost	10%	5	0.50	10	1.0
Key personnel required	10%	8	0.80	10	1.0
Time to complete	10%	8	0.80	10	1.0
Affects other projects	10%	3	0.30	10	1.0
Total			6.30		5.95

Source: Niven, P. R. 2002. "Balanced Scorecard Step by Step," Figure 7.2, *Prioritizing Balanced Scorecard Initiatives,* p. 194, John Wiley & Sons, Inc. Used with permission.

cost, scope, and performance. A successful project will have a scope that specifies the resulting performance level, how much time it will take, and its budgeted cost. A change in any one of these factors will affect the other three.

Exhibit 6.3 demonstrates these relationships graphically. Here, the area of the triangle is a measure of the scope of the project. The length of each side of the triangle indicates the amount of time, money, or performance needed for the project. Because each side of the triangle is connected, changing any of these parameters affects the others. Exhibit 6.4 shows this same project with an increase in required performance level and shortened timelines. Although it has the same scope, this "new" project will incur additional costs.

Although it is difficult to specifically and exactly determine the relationship between all four factors, the successful project manager understands this general relationship well and communicates it to project sponsors. A useful analogy is a balloon: If you push hard on part of it, a different part will bulge out. The classic project management dilemma is an increase in scope without additional time or funding (sometimes termed "scope creep"). Many project failures are directly attributable to ignoring this unyielding formula.

The Project Manager

In most healthcare organizations today, project managers also have other responsibilities. Therefore, it is incumbent on senior management to

Exhibit 6.3
Relationship of
Project Scope to
Performance
Level, Time, and
Cost

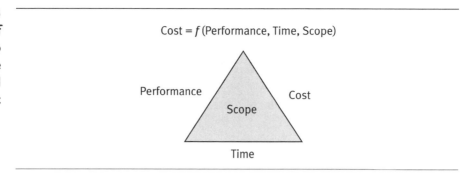

Cost = *f* (Performance, Time, Scope)

Performance   Scope   Cost

Time

Exhibit 6.4
Project with
Increased
Performance
Requirement
and Shortened
Schedule

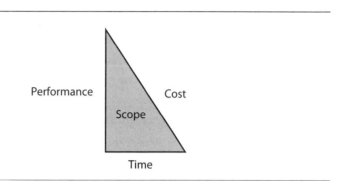

Performance   Scope   Cost

Time

determine how the new responsibility fits with the project manager's current duties and how to reallocate responsibilities if the project manager will be overloaded by taking on the new project.

For clinical projects, it is useful to have dual project managers—a physician leader working closely with an administrator. Most of the project management tasks are accomplished by the administrator, while the physician is involved only in critical clinical issues. For dual project management to work, there must be a strong working relationship between the two. This topic is discussed extensively in Section III of this book.

Stakeholder Identification and Dialogue

The first step in developing a project charter is to identify the stakeholders—in general, anyone who has a stake in the outcome of the project. Key stakeholders include the project manager, customers, users, project team members, any contracted organizations involved, the project sponsor, those who can influence the project, and the project management office.

The project manager is the individual held accountable for the project's success and, therefore, forms the core of the stakeholder group. The customer or user of the service or product is an important stakeholder who will influence and help determine the performance of the final product. Even if project team members have a limited role in the project, its success reflects on them and, therefore, they become stakeholders. A common contracting relationship in healthcare involves large information technology (IT) installations provided through an outside vendor; in such cases, the outside vendor would also be a project stakeholder. A project should always have a sponsor with enough executive-level influence to clear roadblocks as the project progresses; hence, such individuals need to be included in the stakeholder group. A project may be aided or hindered by many individuals or organizations that are not directly part of it, so an effort should be made to identify which of these should be included as stakeholders.

Once stakeholders have been identified, they need to be interviewed by the project manager as he develops the project charter. If an important stakeholder is not available, the project manager should interview someone who represents that person's interests. At this point, it is important to differentiate between the stakeholders' needs and wants, and enough detail must be gathered to adequately construct the project charter. When the project team is organized, it need not include all stakeholders, but the team should attempt to meet all stakeholder needs. The project team should also be cognizant of the organization's culture. Chapter 10 explores the impact of organizational culture and employee engagement in depth. Projects that challenge an organization's culture encounter frequent difficulties.

The project charter is the document that formally authorizes and initiates a project. The project charter provides the project manager with the authority to apply organizational resources to project activities. It also forms a partnership between the requesting organization or department and the project team. A project initiator, or sponsor external to the project, issues the charter and signs it to authorize the start of the project.

Feasibility Analysis

An important part of the project charter is determining the project's feasibility. The senior management team should have prioritized the project, so its link to the organization's strategy has likely been made. However, this link should be documented in the feasibility analysis. Operational and technical feasibility should also be examined. For example, if a new clinical project requires the construction of new facilities, this work may impede its execution. An initial schedule should also be created, as the completion deadline may be impossible to meet. Finally, both financial benefit and marketplace demand should be considered here. All elements of the feasibility analysis should be included in the project charter document.

Project Charter Document

The project charter authorizes the project and serves as an executive summary. A formal charter document should be constructed with the following elements:

- Project mission statement
- Project purpose or justification and link to strategic goals
- High-level requirements that satisfy customers, sponsors, and other stakeholders
- Assigned project manager and authority level
- Summary milestones
- Stakeholder influences
- Functional organizations and their participation
- Organizational, environmental, and external assumptions and constraints
- Financial business case, budget, and return on investment (ROI)
- Project sponsor with approval signature

Exhibit 6.5 is the project charter for the VVH Medicare ACE Project. A project charter template is provided on the companion website of this book, ache.org/books/execution.

The initial description of the scope of the project is found in the Requirements, Milestones, and Financial sections of the project charter.

PROJECT SCOPE AND WORK BREAKDOWN

Once a project has been chartered, the detailed work of planning can begin.

Tools

At this point, the project manager should consider acquiring two important tools. The first is the lowest of low tech, the humble three-ring binder. All projects need a continuous record of progress reports, team meetings, approved changes, and so on. A complex project will require many binders,

**Exhibit 6.5
Project Charter
Format**

Medicare Acute Care Episode (ACE) Project

Project Mission Statement

VVH will develop new processes to improve the quality and lower the costs for a selected set of Medicare patient admissions for orthopedic and cardiac conditions, which will be financed by bundled payments from Medicare.

Project Purpose and Justification

As healthcare costs continue to rise, payers are looking to bundled payments as a method to incentivize providers to optimize care. It is expected that bundled payments will increase from all payers. The ACE demonstration allows VVH to develop the capability to succeed in this new payment environment.

High-Level Requirements

For those admissions included in the ACE project, VVH will:

• Reduce readmissions within 30 days by 40%

• Increase quality measures for bundled payments by 20%

• Make or exceed cost target reductions by 5% on all bundled payments

In addition, the key organizational and process elements required for success will be identified in order to succeed with other bundled payment reimbursement systems.

Assigned Project Managers and Authority Level

Phyllis Colson—Surgery Service Director for Surgical DRGs
Beth Jarvis—Cardiac Service Line Director for Cardiac DRGs
Both project managers have the authority to change time, cost, or performance level by up to 10%. Any changes above that level need project sponsor authorizations.

Summary Milestones

The project will commence on January 1, 2011.
Data analysis will be complete by March 4, 2011.
External provider agreements will be in place by May 11, 2011.
Project will go live on July 7, 2011.

Stakeholder Influences

The following stakeholders will influence this project:

• Physicians will want to provide optimal care to patients.

• VVH clinical staff will want to develop systems for high-quality and cost-effective care.

Continued

but they will prove to be invaluable to the project manager. The classic organization of the binders is by date, so the first pages will be the project charter. Of course, if the organization has an effective imaging and document management system, it can substitute for the binders.

Stakeholder Influences (continued)

- Patients will be interested in and rewarded for participating in the project.
- Vendors will be interested in providing cost-effective solutions for orthopedic and cardiac care.
- VVH financial and IT departments will provide support and analysis through the project and after its go-live date.
- External providers will want to be part of the care continuum for these patients.

Functional Organizations and Their Participation

- Medical directors for orthopedic and cardiac services—leadership
- Inpatient nursing leadership—project management
- Inpatient nurse leaders for orthopedic and cardiac services—participation
- Purchasing (clinical services)—participation
- Finance—participation—financial analysis
- IT—business intelligence and operations—analysis and participation in making changes in EHR

Organizational, Environmental, and External Assumptions and Constraints

- Success depends on changing care patterns consistently by all providers in order to improve quality and decrease cost.
- Providers and vendors who are external to VVH must fully engage and support the project.
- Medicare must make reasonable and consistent payments over the life of the project.

Financial Business Case—Return on Investment (ROI)

Based on other health systems' experience in the ACE project, the following shared savings (additional income) were targeted:

Cardiac DRGs—$650/admission

Orthopedic DRGs—$430/admission

The additional cost for physician supervision, case management, and IT support is $280/admission for both cardiac and orthopedics.

Project Sponsor with Approval Signature

Dr. Moscone, Medical Director

Ira Moscone, MD

The second tool is project management software. Although many options are available, the market leader is Microsoft Project, which is referred to throughout the remainder of the chapter. Microsoft Project is part of the Microsoft Office suite and may already be installed on many computers. If not, a demonstration copy can be downloaded from Microsoft. The companion website for *Healthcare Operations Management* provides additional explanation and videos related to the use of Microsoft Project. (Go to ache.org/books/execution to view a series of videos on the use of Microsoft Project.)

Project management software is not essential for small projects, but it is helpful and almost required for any project that lasts longer than six months and involves a large team of individuals.

Scope

The starting point for developing a scope document is the project charter, although the scope statement is more detailed than the description contained in the project charter. The project manager revisits many of the same stakeholders to acquire more detailed inputs and requirements. A simple methodology is to interview stakeholders and ask them to list the three most important outcomes of the project; these outcomes are then combined with other stakeholders' outcomes and turned into project objectives. It is important that objectives be specific, achievable, measurable, and comprehensible to stakeholders. In addition, they should be stated in terms of time-limited "deliverables." The objective "improve the quality of care to diabetes patients" is a poor one. "Improve the rate of foot exams from baseline by 25 percent in one year for diabetes patients" is better.

It is also important to avoid expanding the scope of the project: "While we are at it, we might as well _____." These ideas, sometimes called "gold plating," tend to be some of the most dangerous in the world of project management. The scope document should also provide detailed requirements and descriptions of expected outcomes. A good scope document also specifies project boundaries—what is inside the project and what is not addressed by the project.

The scope document should specify deliverables, such as implementation of a new process, installation of a new piece of equipment, or presentation of a paper report. The project organization is also specified in the scope document, including the project manager, team members, and specific relationships to all parts of the organization.

An initial evaluation of potential risks to the project should be enumerated in the scope document. The schedule length and milestones should be more detailed in the scope statement than in the charter. As discussed in the next section, however, the final schedule will be developed on the basis of the work breakdown structure. Finally, the scope document should include methods to monitor progress, make changes where necessary, and secure the formal approvals required.

Work Breakdown Structure

The second major component of the scope document is the work breakdown structure, which is considered the engine of the project because it determines how the project goals will be accomplished. The WBS lists the tasks that need to be accomplished, including an estimate of the resources required (e.g., staff time, services, and equipment). For complex projects, the WBS is a hierarchy of major tasks, subtasks, and work packages. Exhibit 6.6 depicts the WBS graphically.

The size of each task should be constructed carefully. A task should not be so small that monitoring would consume a disproportionate share of the task itself. However, an overly large task cannot be effectively monitored and should be divided into subtasks and work packages. The task should have enough detail associated with it that the individual responsible, the cost, and the duration can be identified. A reasonable guideline is that a task should have a duration of one to three weeks to be monitored.

The completion of some tasks is critical to the success of the project. These tasks should be identified as "milestones." The completion of milestones is a convenient shorthand method to communicate overall project progress to stakeholders.

The WBS can be developed by the project team or with the help of outside experts who have executed similar projects. At this point in the project, the WBS is the best estimate of how the project will be executed. It is almost always inaccurate in some way, so the formal control and change procedures described in the following pages are essential to successful project management.

After the WBS has been constructed, the resources required and estimated time for each element must be determined. Estimating the time a task will require is an art. It is best done by a team of individuals. Any previous experiences and data can be helpful.

After a number of meetings, the VVH team determined that the ACE project included three major tasks, each with two subtasks that needed to be accomplished to meet the goals of the project, for a total of six subtasks:

- Acquire external provider data and integrate them into the VVH data warehouse
- Do performance reporting and data mining on the appropriate DRGs and related bundled payment groups to understand current performance
- Use medical staff, benchmarking, literature reviews, and other sources to identify opportunities for improvement

Exhibit 6.6
General WBS
Format

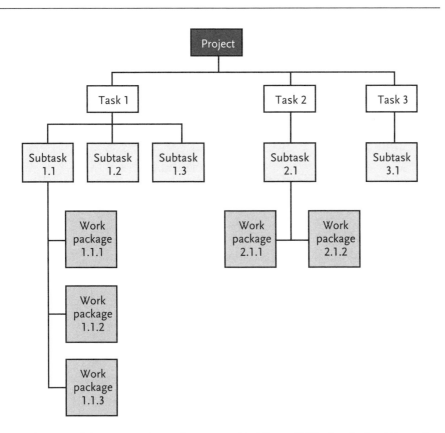

Note: This type of diagram can be easily generated in Microsoft Word and other Microsoft Office products by using the commands Insert → Picture → Organization Chart.

- Solicit cooperation and new relationships with clinicians outside of the VVH system who provided care for VVH-admitted patients
- Revise the EHR to add clinical decision support modules as part of each bundled payment group and targeted DRG
- Convene meetings to educate clinical staff (physicians, nursing, ancillary departments), and modify care guidelines on the basis of their responses

The WBS is displayed in Exhibit 6.7. For a project of this scope to proceed effectively, many more subtasks, perhaps 50 to 100, would be required; in this text, the WBS has been limited to higher-level tasks.

The time estimate for each task is the total time needed to accomplish a task, not the calendar time it will take—a three-day task can be accomplished in three days by one person or in one day by three people.

Exhibit 6.7 WBS for ACE Project

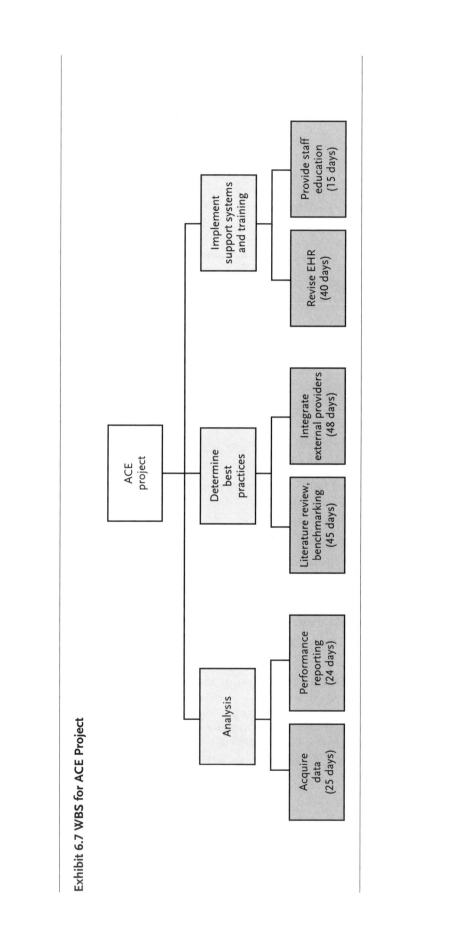

Project Team

The next step is to determine what resources are needed to accomplish these tasks. At VVH, two separate teams were formed—one for cardiac and one for orthopedics. The orthopedic team included[2]

- Phyllis Colson, nursing director for surgery—project manager;
- Karen Bluhm, chief nursing officer;
- Dr. Terry McCollum, chief of orthopedics;
- Sameer Inampudi, director of business intelligence;
- Aaron Martin, director of IT operations; and
- Betty O'Neill, purchasing and outreach.

At this point in the project initiation, it is important to consider the time commitments of all project team members. As opposed to other industries, healthcare organizations do not normally employ full-time project managers. Existing employees are given project management responsibilities in addition to their other job functions. A common mistake is to assign an existing manager and team members with project responsibilities but not relieve other portions of their workload. For projects to succeed, the project manager must have adequate time and resources to successfully execute all of the steps in this formal project management system.

Team members should be clear about their accountability for each task. A functional responsibility chart (sometimes called a RASIC chart) is helpful; the RASIC chart for the ACE project is displayed in Exhibit 6.8. The RASIC diagram is a matrix of team members and tasks from the WBS. For each task, one individual is responsible (R) for ensuring that the task is completed. Other team members may need to approve (A) the completion of the task. Additional team members may work on the task as well, so they are considered support (S). The obligation to inform (I) other team members helps a team communicate effectively. Finally, some team members need to be consulted (C) as a task is being implemented.

SCHEDULING

Network Diagrams and Gantt Charts

Because the WBS was developed without a specific sequence, the next step is scheduling each task to accomplish the total project. First, the logical order of the tasks must be determined. For example, the ACE project team

Exhibit 6.8
RASIC Chart for
ACE Project

WBS Task	Phyllis Colson	Dr. Terry McCollum	Karen Bluhm	Sameer Inampudi	Aaron Martin	Betty O'Neill
Acquire data	A	C	C	R	I	S
Performance reporting	S	A	I	R	C	I
Literature review	R	A	C	I	I	I
Integrate existing providers	C	A	C	I	I	R
Revise EHR	A	C	C	C	R	I
Staff education	R	A	S	I	S	I

R = responsible; A = approval; S = support; I = inform; C = consult.

determined that it needs to acquire a full data set (with data from both internal and external providers) before complete performance reporting and analysis can begin. Other constraints must also be considered, including required start or completion dates and resource availability.

Two tools are used to visually display the schedule. The first is a network diagram that connects each task in order of precedence. A practical way to develop an initial network diagram is to place each task on a sticky note and begin arranging the notes on a set of flip charts until they meet the logical and date constraints. The tasks can then be entered into a project management software system.

Exhibit 6.9 is the network diagram developed by the team for the ACE project. This schedule can be entered into Microsoft Project to generate a similar diagram.

Another common scheduling tool is the Gantt chart, which lists each task on the left side of the page with a bar indicating the start and end times. The Gantt chart for the ACE project, generated by Microsoft Project, is shown in Exhibit 6.10. Each bar indicates the duration of the task, and the small arrows connecting the bars indicate the predecessor–successor relationship of the tasks.

A final review of this initial schedule is done to assess how many tasks are being performed in parallel (simultaneously). A project with few parallel tasks will take longer to accomplish than one with many parallel tasks. Another consideration may be date constraints. Examples include a task that cannot begin until a certain date because of staff availability, or a task that must be completed by a certain date to meet an externally imposed

Exhibit 6.9
Network
Diagram for
ACE Project

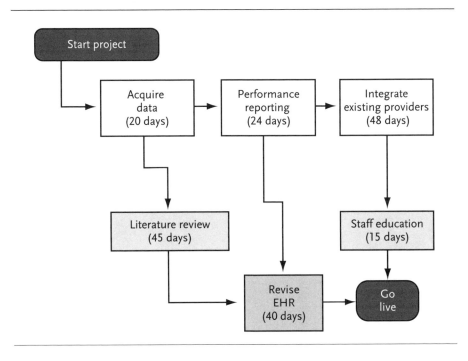

deadline (e.g., new Medicare billing policy). The Project software provides tools to set these constraints in the schedule.

Slack and the Critical Path

To optimize a schedule, the project manager must pay attention to "slack" in the schedule and to the "critical path." If a task takes three days but does not need to be completed for five days, there would be two days of slack. The critical path is the longest sequence of tasks with no slack, or the shortest possible completion time of the project.

Slack is determined by the early finish and late finish dates. The *early finish date* is the earliest date a task could possibly be completed; it is based on the early finish dates of predecessors. The *late finish date* is the latest date a task could be completed without delaying the finish of the project; it is based on the late start and late finish dates of successor tasks. The difference between early finish and late finish dates determines the amount of slack. For critical path tasks (which have no slack), the early finish and late finish dates are identical. Tasks with slack can start later; this later start date is based on the amount of slack available. In other words, if a task takes three days and the earliest the task could be completed is day 18 (as demonstrated by its predecessors), and the late finish date is day 30 (as demonstrated by its successors), the slack for this task is 12 days. This task could start as late as day 27 without affecting the completion date of

Exhibit 6.10 ACE Project Gantt Chart

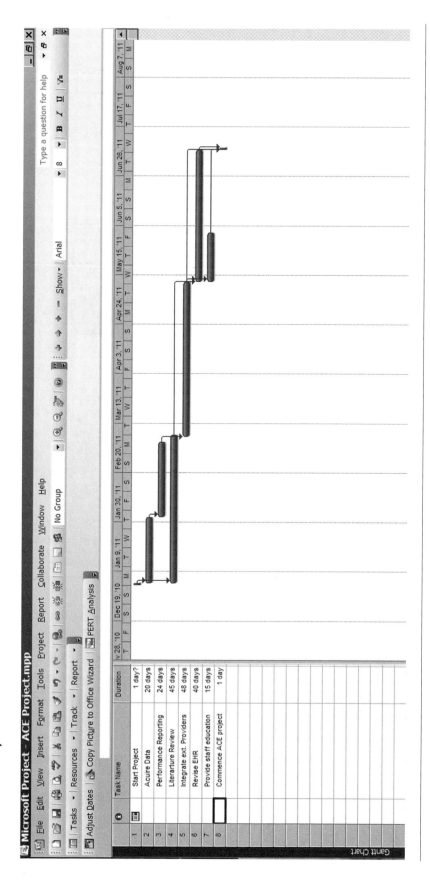

the project. The critical path, which determines the duration of a project, is the connected path through a project of critical tasks.

Exhibit 6.11 displays a Gantt chart for the ACE project with both slack and critical path calculated.

Crashing the Project

Consider the following scenario. VVH has been notified by Medicare that if the ACE project is implemented by June 1, the shared savings funding available to VVH will be increased by 10 percent. Karen Bluhm asks the project manager, Phyllis Colson, to consider speeding up, or "crashing," the project.

The term *project crashing* has negative connotations, as the thought of a computer crashing stirs up dire images. However, a crashed project is simply one that has been sped up. Crashing a project requires reducing the length of the critical path, which can be done by

- shortening the duration of work on a task on the critical path,
- changing a task constraint to allow for more scheduling flexibility,
- breaking a critical task into smaller tasks that can be worked on simultaneously by different resources,
- revising task dependencies to allow more scheduling flexibility,
- setting lead time between dependent tasks where applicable,
- scheduling overtime,
- assigning additional resources to work on critical-path tasks, and
- lowering performance goals (not recommended without strong stakeholder consultation) (Microsoft Office Project Professional Help Screens 2003).

The scope, time, duration, and performance relationships need to be considered in a crashed project. A crashed project has a high risk of costing more than the original schedule predicted, so the formal change procedure discussed in the next section should be used. If the duration of the "integrate providers" task is reduced to 34 days and the "revise EHR" task to 28 days, the project can go live on June 1, 2011.

PROJECT CONTROL

It would be convenient if every project's schedule and costs kept with the initial project plan. Because they almost never do, an effective project

Exhibit 6.11 Gantt Chart for ACE Project with Slack and Critical Path Calculated

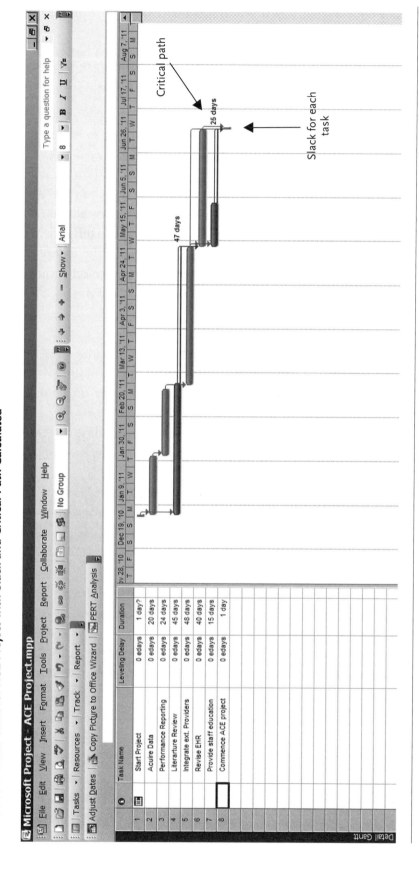

monitoring and change control system needs to be operating throughout the life of a project.

Monitoring Progress

The first important monitoring element is a system that measures schedule completion, cost, and expected performance against the initial plan. Microsoft Project provides a number of tools to assist the project manager with these measures. After the plan's initial scope document, WBS, staffing, and budget have been determined, they are saved as the "baseline plan." Any changes during the project can be compared to this initial baseline.

On a disciplined time basis (e.g., once per week), the project manager needs to receive a progress report from each task manager—the individual designated as "responsible" on the RASIC chart (Exhibit 6.8)—regarding schedule completion and cost. The enterprise version of Project contains some helpful tools to automate this sometimes tedious data gathering task. Exhibit 6.12 shows a Project report on the progress of the ACE project after three weeks.

Note that some preliminary work has begun on the performance reporting task, even though the acquire data task is not complete. This parallel processing can help make up for unexpected delays later in the project.

Change Control

The project manager should have a status meeting at least once a month, and preferably more frequently. At this meeting, the project team should review the status of the project on the basis of task completion, expenses, personnel utilization, and progress toward expected project outcomes. The majority of time in these meetings should be devoted to problem solving, not reporting.

Once deviations are detected, the team must determine their sources and causes. Three courses of action are available: Ignore the deviation if it is small, take corrective action to remedy the problem, or modify the plan by using the formal change procedure developed in the project charter and scope document.

Events that occur outside the project are one major cause of deviations. The environment will always be changing during a project's execution, and modifications of the project's scope or performance level may be necessary.

Exhibit 6.12 Status of ACE Project at Three Weeks

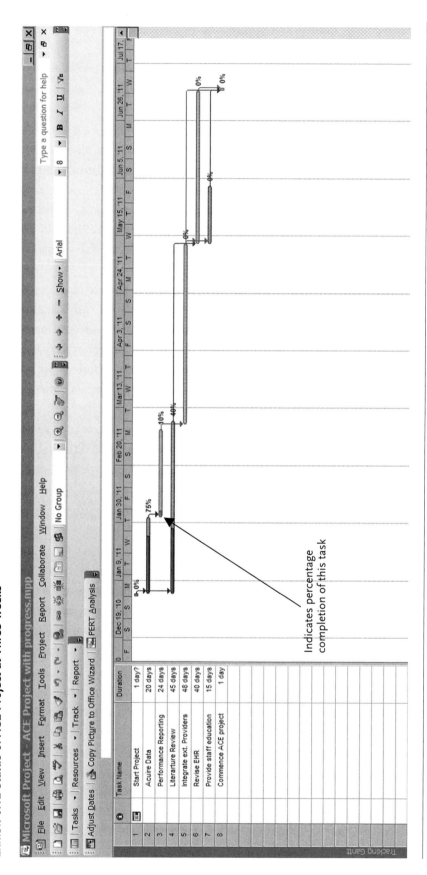

For example, if a competitor initiates a new service, the hospital may change its project scope to respond.

High-performing project managers understand the importance of using a formal change mechanism. It is human nature to resist communicating a schedule or cost problem to project sponsors and stakeholders. However, the consequences of this inaction can be significant, if not fatal, to large projects. The change process also forces all parties involved in a project to subject themselves to disciplined analysis of options and creates disincentives for scope creep. Changes to the initial plan should be documented in writing, approved by the project sponsor as appropriate, and included in the project records (three-ring binders or equivalent).

The ACE project charter (and subsequent scope document) states that changes of less than 10 percent can be made by project manager Phyllis Colson. Therefore, she could adjust the schedule by up to 10.3 days and the shared savings goal by $43 per admission. For deviations greater than these amounts, Colson would need the approval of the project sponsor (Dr. Moscone).

COMMUNICATIONS

A formal communications plan was developed as part of scope creation. Communications to both internal and external stakeholders are critical to the success of a project. Many media can be used, including oral briefings, e-mail, and formal reports. Many organizations establish a Web-based intranet that contains detailed information on the project. An e-mail is sent to stakeholders periodically, with a summary progress report and links back to the website for more detailed information. A sophisticated system communicates only issues of interest to each stakeholder. As part of the communications strategy, feedback from stakeholders should always be solicited, as changes in the project plan may be affecting the stakeholder in ways unknown to the project manager.

Project update communications should contain information gathered from quantitative reports. At a minimum, these communications should provide progress against baseline on schedule, cost, scope, and expected performance. Any changes to project baseline, as well as the approval process, should be noted. Any issues that need resolution, or those that are being resolved, should also be noted. The expected completion date is always of interest to all stakeholders and should be a prominent part of any project plan communication.

RISK MANAGEMENT

Comprehensive prospective risk management is another component of successful projects. A *risk* is an event that will cause the project to deviate substantially from planned schedule, cost, scope, or performance. Like many other aspects of project management, it takes discipline to develop a risk management plan at the beginning of a project and to update it continuously as the project progresses.

The most direct way to develop a risk management plan is to begin with the WBS. Each task in the WBS should be assessed for risks. Each task is subject to risk in performance, duration, or cost; if a project has 50 tasks, it has 150 potential risks.

A number of techniques can be used to identify risks, but the most straightforward is a brainstorming exercise by the project team. (Some of the tools found in *Healthcare Operations Management* Chapter 6—e.g., mind mapping, root cause analysis, force field analysis—could also be used in risk assessment.) Another useful technique is to interview stakeholders and ask them what risks they perceive. The organization's strategic plan is also a resource. If the plan was developed using the Design and Planning School approach (see Chapter 2), it will contain a strengths, weaknesses, opportunities, and threats (SWOT) analysis. The weaknesses and threats sections may contain clues to potential risks to a project task.

Once risks have been identified for each task in the WBS structure, the project team should assign a risk probability to each. The risks with the highest probability (i.e., likelihood of occurring during the project) should be analyzed in depth. A risk management strategy should be devised to deal with each.

Tasks with the following characteristics should be looked at closely, as they may be high risk:

- Of long duration
- Subject to highly variable estimates of duration
- Dependent on external organizations
- Dependent on a unique resource (e.g., a physician who is on call)
- Likely to be affected by external governmental or payer policies

The management strategy for each identified risk should have three components. First, risk prevention initiatives should be identified. It is always better to avoid an adverse event than to have to deal with its consequences. An example of a risk prevention strategy is to provide mentoring to a young team member who is responsible for key tasks in the project plan.

The second element of the risk management strategy is a mitigation plan. An example of a mitigation response would be to bring additional people and financial resources to a task. Another might be to call on the project sponsor to help break an organizational logjam.

Third, a project team may decide to transfer the risk by purchasing insurance against the risk. This strategy is common in construction projects through the use of bonding for contractors.

All identified risks and their management plans should be outlined in a *risk register*—a listing of each task, identified risks, and prevention and mitigation plans. This risk management plan should be updated throughout the life of the project.

The ACE project team identified three serious risks, which are listed in Exhibit 6.13 with their mitigation plans.

QUALITY MANAGEMENT, PROCUREMENT, AND PROJECT CLOSURE

Quality Management

The majority of focus in this chapter has been on managing the scope, cost, and schedule of a project. The performance, or quality, of an operational project is the fourth key element in successful project management. In general, *quality* is defined as meeting specified performance levels with minimal variation and waste.

A complete discussion of quality management is beyond the scope of this book and can be found in *Healthcare Operations Management*, chapters 6, 8, and 9.

Throughout the life of a project, the project team should monitor the expected quality of the final product. Individual tasks that are part of a quality management function within a project should be created in the WBS. For example, the revisions to the EHR may include clinical decision support modules that support clinical staff in providing optimal care and meeting the clinical quality goals for the project.

Procurement

Many projects depend on outside vendors and contractors, so a procurement system integrated with an organization's project management system is essential. A purchasing or procurement department can be helpful

Exhibit 6.13
Risk Mitigation
Plan for ACE
Project

Risk	Mitigation Plan
Acquiring data is complex due to varied data systems of external providers.	Assistance will be sought from an external data integration vendor who will be contracted and used as necessary.
Integration of external providers is difficult due to financial expectations of these providers.	An RFP will be created and issued. External providers will therefore understand financial and performance expectations.
Software modifications to EHR are more expensive than budgeted.	Contingency funding has been earmarked in the VVH IT budget.

in this process. Procurement staff will have developed templates for many of the processes described in the next sections. They will also have knowledge of the latest legal constraints an organization may face. However, the most useful attribute of the procurement department may be the frequency with which it executes the purchasing cycle. By performing this task frequently, its staff have developed expertise in the process and are aware of common pitfalls.

Contracting

Once an organization has decided to contract with a vendor for a portion of a project, three basic types of contracting are available. The *fixed-price contract* is a lump sum for the performance of specified tasks. Fixed-price contracts sometimes include incentives for early delivery.

Cost reimbursement contracts provide the vendor a payment based on the vendor's direct and indirect costs of delivering the service for a specified task. It is important to clearly document in advance how the vendor will calculate its costs.

The most open-ended type of contract is known as *time and materials*. Here, the task itself may be poorly defined, and the contractor is reimbursed for her actual time, materials, and overhead. A time and materials–type contract is commonly used for remodeling an older building, where the contractor is not certain of what she will find in the walls. Great caution and monitoring are needed when an organization uses this type of contracting.

All contracts should contain a statement of work (SOW). The SOW contains a detailed scope statement, including WBS, for the work that will be performed by the contractor. It also includes expected quantity and quality levels, performance data, task durations, work locations, and other details that will be used to monitor the work of the contractor.

Selecting a Vendor

Once a preliminary SOW has been developed, the organization will solicit proposals and select a vendor. A useful first step is to issue a request for information (RFI) to as many possible vendors as the project team can identify. The RFIs generate responses from vendors about their products and experience with similar organizations. On the basis of these responses, the number of feasible vendors can be reduced to a manageable set.

A more formal request for proposal (RFP) can then be issued. The RFP will ask for a detailed proposal, or bid. The following criteria should be considered in awarding the contract:

- Does the vendor clearly understand the organization's requirements?
- What is the total cost?
- Does the vendor have the capability and correct technical approach to deliver the requested service?
- What is the vendor's management approach to monitoring execution of the SOW?
- Can the vendor provide maintenance or meet future requirements and changes?
- Can the vendor provide references that are similar to the contracting organization?
- Does the vendor assert intellectual or proprietary property rights in the products it supplies?

Project Closure

A successful project should have an organized closure process, which includes a formal stakeholder presentation and approval process. In addition, the project sponsor should sign off at project completion to signify that performance levels have been achieved and all deliverables have been received. During the closeout process, special attention should be paid to project staff, who will be interested in their next assignment. A disciplined handoff of staff from one project to the next will complete the closure process.

All documents related to the project should be indexed and stored. Archives can be helpful if outside vendors have participated in the project and a contract dispute arises. Historical documents also can provide a good starting point for the next version of a project.

The project team should have a final session to identify lessons learned—both good and bad—in the execution of the project. These lessons should be included in the project documentation and shared with other project managers in the organization.

THE PROJECT MANAGER AND PROJECT TEAM

The project manager's role is pivotal to the success of any project. Selecting, developing, and nurturing high-functioning team members are also critical. The project manager's team skills include running effective meetings and facilitating optimal dialogue during these meetings.

A project manager can take on many roles. In some smaller healthcare projects, the project manager is actually the person who accomplishes many of the project tasks. In other projects, the project manager's job is solely leadership and management of the individuals performing the tasks.

Team Structure and Authority

The members and structure of a project team may be selected by the project manager, but in many cases the project sponsor and other members of senior management make these decisions. It is important to formally document the team makeup and how team members were assigned in the project charter and scope documents. Care should be taken to avoid over-scheduling team members, as all members must have the needed time available to work on the project.

A number of key issues need to be addressed as the project team is formed. The most important is the project manager's level of authority to make decisions. Can the project manager commit resources, or must she ask senior management or department heads each time a new resource is needed? Is the budget controlled by the project manager, or does a central financial authority control it? Finally, is administrative support available to the team, or do the project team members need to perform these tasks themselves?

Team Meetings

A weekly or biweekly project team meeting is highly recommended to keep a project on schedule. At this meeting, the project's progress can be monitored and discussed, and actions to resolve deviations and problems can be initiated.

All good team meetings include comprehensive agendas and a complete set of minutes. Minutes should be action oriented (e.g., "The schedule slippage for task 17 will be resolved by assigning additional resources from the temporary pool"). In addition, the individual accountable for following through on the issue should be identified. If the meeting's deliberations and actions are confidential, everyone on the team should be aware of this policy and adhere to it uniformly.

The decision-making process should be clear and understood by all team members. In some situations, all major decisions will be made by the project manager. In others, team members may have veto power if they represent a major department that may need to commit new resources. Some major decisions may need to be reviewed and approved by individuals external to the project team. The use of data and analytical techniques is strongly encouraged as a part of the decision process.

Team members need to take responsibility for the success of the team. They can demonstrate this behavior by following through on commitments, contributing to the discussion, actively listening, and giving and accepting feedback. Everyone on a team should feel that she has a voice, and the project manager needs to lead the meeting in such a way as to balance the "air time" between team members. This means politely and artfully interrupting long-winded team members and summarizing their points; it also means calling on silent team members to solicit input.

At the end of a meeting, it is useful to evaluate the meeting itself. The project manager and team can spend a few minutes reviewing these and other questions:

- Did we accomplish our purpose?
- Did we take steps to maintain our gains?
- Did we document actions, results, and ideas?
- Did we work together successfully?
- Did we share our results with others?
- Did we recognize everyone's contribution and celebrate our achievements?

The performance of project teams is affected by the organization's leaders and the organizational culture. These forces are explored more comprehensively in Section III of this book.

THE PROJECT MANAGEMENT OFFICE

Many organizations outside the healthcare industry (e.g., architects, consultants) are primarily project oriented. Such organizations have a centralized project management office (PMO) to oversee the work of their staff. Because healthcare delivery organizations are primarily operational, the majority do not use this structure.

However, departments in large hospitals and clinics, such as IT and quality, have begun to use a centralized project office approach. In addition, some organizations have designated and trained project leaders in Six Sigma or Lean techniques. These project leaders are assigned from a central PMO.

PMOs provide a central structure from which to monitor progress on all projects in an organization and reallocate resources as needed when projects encounter problems. They also provide a resource for the training and development of project managers. PMOs support project managers by (Project Management Institute 2008)

- managing shared resources;
- developing project management methodology, best practices, and standards;
- coaching, mentoring, training, and providing oversight;
- developing and managing policies, procedures, templates, and other shared documentation;
- monitoring compliance with standards, policies, procedures, and templates; and
- coordinating communication.

Another useful function for a PMO is to maintain an information system that can provide reports to project stakeholders and senior management. The contents of this information system can include

- progress reports on individual projects (schedule, cost, performance),
- risk management information (high-risk tasks and their current status),
- documentation on performance failures and remediation steps, and
- a log of lessons learned.

Bob Olson (COO of VVH) felt that it was important to establish a PMO if all the initiatives he had on his plate were to be executed effectively. Chapter 7 provides a description of the VVH PMO.

SUMMARY

This chapter provides an introduction to the science and discipline of formal project management. The probability of successfully carrying out a project that will meet the schedule, budget, and performance requirements increases significantly if the formal PMI project management methodology is used. Key components of this system include the project charter, stakeholder analysis, WBS and schedule, project software for monitoring and critical-path analysis, effective project communications, and disciplined risk control and change management.

Special attention needs to be paid to the creation, function, and staffing of the project team. A PMO can be created to centrally support and monitor all projects in an organization.

NOTES

1. A recent review of the scientific basis for project management has been conducted by Carden and Egan. They found that "refereed research has indicated that project managers utilize tools and techniques along with people to ensure quality deliverables are on time, within scope, and within budget. Additionally, project leadership and a favorable development environment both are important to the successful delivery of projects. Therefore, there is a connection between knowledge and action that can be used to frame behaviors by engaging in transactions to plan, organize, monitor, and report findings in order to maintain a dynamic balance with the organization, resources, tools, and the external environment" (Carden and Egan 2008).

2. For the remainder of this chapter, only the orthopedic portion of this project will be detailed.

Variations on Project Management and Clinical Innovation

THE PROJECT MANAGEMENT Institute (PMI) approach to project management, described in Chapter 6, has a high probability of producing expected results. However, it is complex and requires skilled project managers.

A number of other approaches and variations on this methodology have been developed. They are focused on three types of projects: (1) smaller projects, (2) projects whose specific tasks are not known at the outset, and (3) process improvement projects.

This chapter will therefore provide an overview of

- agile project management,
- Lean Six Sigma and the DMAIC project model,
- the IHI model for improvement, and
- a comparison of all project management approaches.

In addition, the specific case of clinical innovation and its future will be addressed.

STATE OF THE ART

Agile Project Management

In some situations, knowledge of the tasks necessary for project success is not available as the project is chartered and scheduled. In these cases, agile project management often works better than other methods. Agile project management is "adaptive," in contrast to the "predictive" style of formal project management.

Agile project management has a number of characteristics:

- Customer satisfaction is achieved by rapid, continuous delivery of services or new processes.
- Newly prototyped services or processes are delivered frequently (weekly rather than monthly).
- The effectiveness and ease of use of these prototypes are the principal measures of progress.
- Late changes to requirements are welcome.
- There is close, daily cooperation between customers and the project team.
- Face-to-face conversation is the best form of communication (co-location).
- There is continuous attention to technical excellence and good design in the new services or processes.
- There is regular adaptation to changing circumstances.

Exhibit 7.1 illustrates agile project management.

Agile project management is best used for "mysteries" to which there are no known answers (e.g., finding the best treatment for a new emerging disease) as opposed to "puzzles" to which the answer is known but complex (e.g., building a new clinic).

Lean Six Sigma and DMAIC

Process improvement is a known science practiced in many industries and is now becoming widely used in progressive healthcare organizations. The most common approach used currently by many organizations is Lean Six Sigma.

Lean Six Sigma is a combination of two streams of process improvement approaches. The Lean enterprise approach to process improvement improves flow and eliminates waste. Six Sigma has roots in statistical process control; its main goal is to refine processes to produce highly reliable and predictable results. Many practitioners have combined the best of both approaches into Lean Six Sigma. The details of these methodologies are beyond the scope of this book; a comprehensive review with many examples is contained in *Healthcare Operations Management*.

Exhibit 7.1
Agile Project
Management

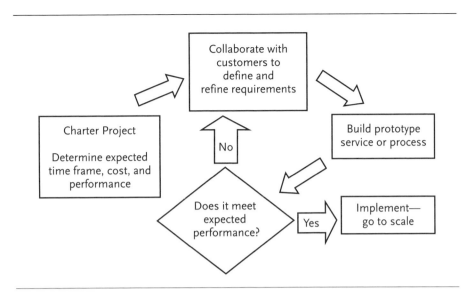

The Lean Six Sigma project management approach is summarized in the acronym DMAIC. This system originated from the Six Sigma methodology. Each project includes five major steps:

1. Define

In the define phase, the Six Sigma project team chooses a project on the basis of the business's strategic objectives and the requirements of the process's customers. The problem to be solved (or process to be improved) is defined in terms of measurable results. "Good" Six Sigma projects typically have the following attributes:

- The project will save or make money for the organization.
- The desired process outcomes are measurable.
- The problem is important to the business, has a clear relationship to organizational strategy, and is (or will be) supported by the organization.

In the define phase, internal and external customers of the process are identified and their "critical to quality" (CTQ) characteristics are determined. CTQ characteristics are the key measurable characteristics of a product or process for which minimum performance standards desired by the customer can be determined.

2. Measure

In the measure phase, the team determines the current capability and stability of the process. The inputs to the process, as well as the key process input and output variables, are identified and prioritized. The purpose of this phase of the project is to establish the current state of the process so that the effect of any process changes can be evaluated.

3. Analyze

In the analyze phase, the team analyzes the data that have been collected to determine the root causes or key process input variables. This analysis helps the team decide how best to eliminate variation or failure in the process and improve the outcomes. In some cases, powerful statistical tools are used to analyze and understand the underlying causes of poor performance in a system.

4. Improve

In the improve phase, the team identifies, evaluates, and implements the improvement solutions. Possible solutions are identified and evaluated in terms of their probability of successful implementation. A plan for deployment of solutions is developed, and the solutions are implemented. Actual results are measured to quantify the effect of the project.

5. Control

In the control phase, controls are put in place to ensure process improvement gains are maintained and that the process does not revert to the "old way." The improvements are institutionalized through modification of structures and systems (e.g., training, incentives, monitoring).

Kaizen and Rapid Process Improvement Workshops

The Lean methodology does not have a significant project management structure. Instead, it supports large-scale change through many short process improvement events. These "kaizen" events are focused on immediate process analysis and improvement. They are also known as Rapid Process Improvement Workshops (RPIWs) and usually take between one and five days. RPIWs can be identified as tasks that are parts of larger and more complex projects.

IHI Model for Improvement

The Institute for Healthcare Improvement (IHI) continues to be a national leader in clinical quality improvement. As part of this leadership, IHI has developed a straightforward project improvement model. The model includes five major steps:

1. Set Aims

The first step is to establish aims that are time specific and measurable. In addition, they should define the specific patients who will be affected. "Reduce incidence of ventilator-associated pneumonia by 25 percent" is an example of a critical care aim.

2. Establish Measures

The second step is to establish measures that are more specific than the project aims. They can be outcome, process, or balanced measures (i.e., measures that look at a system from different dimensions) or a combination.

3. Select Changes

To achieve the project's aims, the team must implement change in the current operation environment. At this point, a change method needs to be selected. Change methods include: eliminating waste, improving work flow, optimizing inventory, changing the work environment, changing supply chain relationships, reducing variation, and error proofing.

4. Test Changes

To test an improvement, the team uses the Plan-Do-Study-Act (PDSA) cycle (Exhibit 7.2). The change is planned, it is done, the effect is studied, and the results are acted upon—either the change has been effective or a new change needs to be planned. The PDSA cycle is based on the scientific method and is effective for making specific and long-lasting change.

5. Implement Changes

If a change is proven on a small scale, it probably will be valuable in similar environments. For example, a scheduling system that reduced waiting times in one clinic might be beneficial to all clinics in an integrated healthcare delivery system.

COMPARING AND SELECTING THE PROJECT MANAGEMENT SYSTEM

The choice of project management approach depends on the project scale and clarity of the expected results. Although there is clearly crossover and

Exhibit 7.2
PDSA Change
Methodology

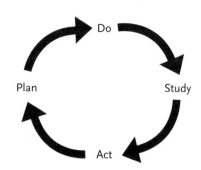

commonality between all of the methods described in this chapter and Chapter 6, a few rules of thumb can be used to make this selection. For large-scale projects that are complex and risky, the PMI formal project management system described in Chapter 6 should be used. For less complex and risky projects, the IHI system is sufficient.

In some cases, the project manager does not know in advance what the result of the project will be because the problem falls into the "mystery" category mentioned earlier. If the case is about improving a specific process, the Lean Six Sigma DMAIC approach should be used. If the process itself is unclear, the agile project management approach should be used. Exhibit 7.3 illustrates how to select these methodologies.

Elements of each system can also be combined. For example, detailed task scheduling (which is part of the PMI approach) can be used in a DMAIC project. The quality measurement tools of DMAIC can be used in an agile project to determine when the product of the project is performing as expected.

In all cases, a project charter needs to be completed and progress needs be tracked and reported. The best way to track progress is through a project management office (PMO).

CLINICAL INNOVATION—REDUCING THE 17 YEARS

It takes 17 years for proven research evidence to be used by 50 percent of physicians (Balas and Boren 2000). This classic finding was published in 2000, and the challenge continues today. Implementing new clinical knowledge in a timely and effective manner must be a priority for all healthcare providers.

Historically, most clinical innovations have been initiated by physicians who are willing to lead improvements. These projects arise from their rigorous reading of medical journals, attendance at conferences in their specialty, courses taken at academic health centers, or a new payer policy

Exhibit 7.3
Selecting Project
Management
Methods

```
                                    ┌──────────────────┐
                          ┌─────────┤                  │
                 Yes      │                            ┌───────────┐
                  ┌───────◇ Complex        ────────────►   PMI     │
                          │ and high                   │           │
                          │ risk      No               └───────────┘
                          ◇       ────────┐
                          ▲               │
                 Yes      │               │            ┌───────────┐
                          │               └────────────►    IHI    │
  ┌──────────┐            ◇ Final                      │           │
  │ Initiate │ ──────────► product                     └───────────┘
  │ project  │            │ known
  └──────────┘            ◇
                          │
                 No       │                            ┌───────────┐
                          │                  ┌─────────►   Agile    │
                          ▼                  │         │           │
                          ◇ Complex   No     │         └───────────┘
                          │ process  ────────┘
                          │ improvement                ┌───────────┐
                          ◇                  ┌──────────►   DMAIC   │
                              Yes            │         │           │
                          └──────────────────┘         └───────────┘
```

that encourages the use of a new treatment or diagnostic procedure. Unfortunately, this system is too haphazard and unpredictable to broadly improve the quality of care. In addition, it does not adequately address the 17-year knowledge-transfer problem.

Organized Clinical Innovation

Progressive healthcare delivery organizations now have an organized clinical innovation process. It includes three basic steps: identifying targets for improvement, chartering and implementing project teams (using one of the methods described in this chapter or Chapter 6), and embedding the innovation (see Chapter 8).

The targets for innovation continue to arise from clinical leaders, but many organizations also use a variety of other sources, including

- publicly reported measures of clinical quality,
- the list of conditions under review for comparative effectiveness by the Agency for Healthcare Research and Quality,

- the IHI Improvement Map,
- the National Quality Forum list of potentially overused services and conditions, and
- the United States Preventive Services Task Force.

A review of these sources will yield a long list of potential projects. This list can be prioritized by ranking each condition relative to its prevalence inside the organization and the size of the current performance gap.

Large-Scale Spread

Implementing clinical change is a challenge in all circumstances but is particularly difficult when the goal is widespread change in clinical practice. IHI pioneered large-scale change with the 100,000 Lives Campaign in 2004. This project achieved its goal of saving more than 100,000 lives of patients who might otherwise have died unnecessarily in hospitals in the United States (Institute for Healthcare Improvement 2006).

To effect large-scale change, improvement teams need to pay significant attention to the environment and culture of the organizations participating in the change. IHI suggests that a number of major factors be managed during large-scale change:

- Motivation—What are the motivation and commitment of the leaders of the change? Is there an urgent need for the change? Is the scale of the change possible?
- Foundation—How does this change effort fit into larger organizational goals and culture? What process of project management will be used? Who will lead it? Who will support it?
- Aim—What are the aim, time frame, and measures?
- Nature of the intervention—How will the change work, and will it be effective?
- Nature of the social system—What is the organization's culture, and will it accept this change? Are the needed resources available, including participants' time?
- Communication and support—How will participants be supported and recognized? How will successes be communicated? What data will be collected and disseminated?

Rapid Learning from Electronic Health Records—The Future

Basic clinical research has led to many innovations in healthcare delivery. The primary tool for validating new findings is the randomized clinical trial. However, even the current state of the art in clinical trials has caused concern. Some of the problems include bias toward younger patients in the trials, few studies that compare different therapies, and wide variations in results among patient subpopulations (Etheredge 2007).

Fortunately, the rise of the electronic health record (EHR) provides an opportunity to advance medical knowledge in a larger context. EHRs can be used to collect and analyze large data sets from real patients to determine which treatments are most effective. In addition, these databases can be used to develop mathematical patient models that simulate the effects of new treatments or drugs without the use of clinical trials. Dr. David Eddy has developed such a model, called Archimedes. In a recent diabetes study, results from the Archimedes model correlated with results from an actual patient study 98 percent of the time (Eddy 2007).

NOTES FROM THE FIELD

HealthPartners

HealthPartners has created a department devoted to care, innovation, and measurement to advance clinical innovation. The department uses a number of inputs to help it charter projects, including Institute of Medicine studies, publicly reported conditions, and Healthcare Effectiveness Data and Information Set (HEDIS) measures. It also focuses on new business lines that have been identified as part of its strategic plans.

HealthPartners' improvement teams comprise 8 to 15 members. They are usually led by a physician and an administrator and receive substantial support from members of the Care, Innovation, and Measurement Department. The teams include members from clinical departments, finance, and IT. In some cases patients are also invited.

Each project is chartered and approved by a sponsor who is a senior leader within HealthPartners. The charter includes four basic sections: (1) outcomes desired, (2) drivers of the outcome, (3) tactics to achieve the outcome, and (4) measures. The Care, Innovation, and Measurement Department develops a preliminary process redesign and improvement plan with the leaders. The project team convenes, and a rapid design session is held over one or two days to review, revise, and tune up the preliminary redesign to be clinically efficient and patient centered.

The new process is piloted in multiple sites, and changes are made on the basis of these preliminary results. Once a final process design has been developed, the leaders determine the most effective methodology to spread the improvement. One example used frequently by HealthPartners is a large, off-site meeting attended by staff from all delivery sites and departments that will be affected by the change. A final tune-up is done, and the new process is implemented throughout HealthPartners. Results are monitored and integrated into HealthPartners' reporting systems and dashboards.

HealthPartners uses the IHI model for improvement and some elements of Lean Six Sigma.

VINCENT VALLEY HEALTHCARE

Accountable Care Organization

The VVH accountable care organization (ACO) team included four care managers, two researchers, and one part-time IT member. It was led by Sally Campion, who was an experienced clinic nurse, most recently from the diabetes center at VVH. She wanted to see if the chronic disease management tools that worked for management of diabetics could be applied to a larger and more diverse population. The team decided to use a combination of PMI-style project management with an agile overlay. The use of agile project management reflected the team's concern that effective disease management is still more of an art than a science than most practitioners would admit.

After the team developed a preliminary work plan and schedule, a formal charter was approved by Bob Olson, COO of VVH. However, a number of the tasks in the schedule had long durations and were considered research projects. These projects were designed to test various disease management approaches that the staff had identified from the literature and from discussions with similar organizations and health plans.

Physical space was important to the ACO project team, so it set up a large open-space office in a building next to VVH hospital. Each team member had an open cubicle and freely discussed ideas and successes with other team members. A whiteboard, used by the team to track experiments and results, completely covered one wall.

Each morning the team huddled for 15 minutes to coordinate the day's work. Once per week, the project schedule was reviewed and revised on the basis of the results of that week's experiments. The initial experiments for post-discharge care included four tasks:

- Follow-up by phone to ensure clinic visits and referrals to specialists
- Consultation with social workers on discharge plans
- Expedited creation of discharge summaries and communications with primary care physicians
- Review of all discharge medications by VVH pharmacists

Once an experiment proved successful for six months, it was considered a new process and was embedded in the clinical decision support system of the VVH EHR.

The Project Management Office

Because of the breadth of the strategic initiatives under way at VVH, Olson felt it was imperative that he establish a PMO. He had two of his younger managers attend training to achieve their PMP certification, and they became the staff of the PMO.

The PMO staff undertook the duties described in Chapter 6, with a special emphasis on ensuring that major projects had charters detailing expected outcomes, schedules, and costs. One challenge was to identify which projects to track centrally, as all good managers have many projects under way at all times. VVH determined that its PMO would track projects that

- were part of the corporate strategy map,
- required a significant capital investment (greater than $500,000),
- were critical to publicly reported quality results,
- were high priorities of the medical staff, and
- could significantly improve financial results.

The PMO staff requested monthly updates from all active projects regarding progress, schedules, and costs. They provided consulting help to projects that were behind or over budget. In addition, they provided a communications link across the organization to ensure that projects were complementary to each other and that synergy and expected outcomes were being achieved organization-wide.

SUMMARY

For complex projects, the PMI formal project management system described in Chapter 6 should be used. However, other project approaches are also useful. The agile project management approach can be used when all tasks in a project are not known at its outset. For projects focused on process improvement, the Lean Six Sigma DMAIC framework is effective. For straightforward clinical projects, the IHI improvement method is relatively simple and practical.

Clinical innovation needs to be more widespread. To this aim, new methods for broad implementation are being tested and implemented. The broad use of the electronic health record will be the vehicle for the rapid spread of clinical innovation in the future.

RESOURCES

- Agency for Healthcare Research and Quality (www.ahrq.gov/clinic/outcomix.htm)
- Institute for Healthcare Improvement
  - Improvement map (www.ihi.org/IHI/Programs/ImprovementMap)
  - IHI project management (www.ihi.org/IHI/Topics/Improvement/ImprovementMethods/HowToImprove)
  - Large-scale spread (www.ihi.org/IHI/Results/WhitePapers/PlanningforScaleWhitePaper.htm)
- National Quality Forum (www.qualityforum.org)
- United States Preventive Services Task Force (www.ahrq.gov/clinic/pocketgd09)
  - Downloads available: project charter templates: Agile, Lean Six Sigma (A3), IHI

CHAPTER 8

Embedding the Change

A WELL-EXECUTED strategy is only effective if it is maintained and improved. Many newly installed processes perform well initially but then drift slowly into an unsatisfactory level of performance. Therefore, it is important in any project plan to include a mechanism to embed the changes and monitor their performance. This chapter will provide an overview of tools to accomplish this task:

- General Systems Theory and the role of feedback
- Operating procedures and process maps
- Checklists
- Control charts
- Dashboards and scorecards
- Automated business rules
- Clinical decision support
- Huddles, transparency, and direct accountability

STATE OF THE ART

General Systems Theory and the Role of Feedback

Adherence to the principles of General Systems Theory will help an organization maintain stability and performance in a new system.

No system is ever completely stable. Each system's performance is modified and controlled by feedback (see exhibits 8.1 and 8.2). Feedback is "any reciprocal flow of influence. In systems thinking it is an axiom that every influence is both *cause* and *effect*" (Senge 1990).

Feedback can be either reinforcing or balancing. *Reinforcing feedback* prompts change that builds on itself and amplifies the outcome of a process, taking the process further and further from its starting point. The effect of reinforcing feedback can be positive or negative. For example, a reinforcing change of positive financial results for an organization could be higher salaries, which could lead to even better financial performance because the pay increase would likely heighten its employees' motivation (see Exhibit 8.1). In contrast, poor supervision could contribute to employee turnover, short staffing, and even more turnover.

Balancing feedback prompts change that seeks stability. A balancing feedback loop attempts to return the system to its starting point (see Exhibit 8.2). For example, a clinical treatment process that controls drug dosing via real-time monitoring of a patient's physiological responses is an example of balancing feedback. Inpatient unit staffing levels that drive the location of a newly admitted hospital patient are another. Both of these feedback mechanisms are designed to maintain balance in the system.

A confounding problem with feedback is delay. Delays occur when there are interruptions between actions and consequences. As a result, systems tend to overshoot and perform poorly. For example, an emergency department might experience a surge in patients and call in additional staff. If this unexpected demand for care subsides quickly, the added staff may not be needed and unnecessary expense will have been incurred. Delays also make controlling and maintaining changes difficult. For example, if an operating room governing committee meets only once per quarter to adjust scheduling, it is likely that the adjustments will slide during the ensuing months due to various surgeons' preferences. A more effective monitoring and feedback system would have this committee meet every other week to review actual data from the most current 14 days and make adjustments if needed.

To embed changes, improvement teams need to understand the systems in which change resides. Every change will be resisted and reinforced by feedback mechanisms, many of which are not clearly visible. Taking a broad systems view can improve the effectiveness of change.

Operating Procedures and Process Maps

Almost all significant executions of strategy involve installing new processes. Two basic tools can help an organization integrate and embed them. The first is the standardized procedure. A written standard operating procedure (SOP) reduces variations in performance among individuals or groups, provides a basis for training new employees, gives directions in unusual cases, and provides

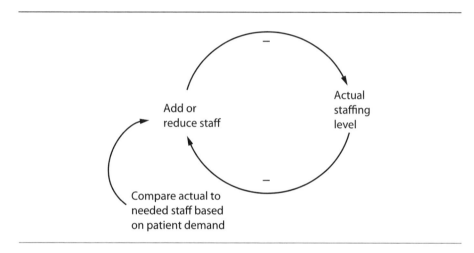

**Exhibit 8.1
System with
Reinforcing
Feedback**

**Exhibit 8.2
System with
Balancing
Feedback**

a trail along which problems can be traced. SOPs should include expected per-formance and cost metrics, and these metrics should be monitored rigorously.

Additional details and logic for a SOP can be provided by a process map (also called a flowchart). A process map is a graphic description of the in-puts, outputs, and steps in a process. Exhibit 8.3 is an example of a process map for patient check-in at a clinic. (A more detailed description of process mapping and improvement is available in *Healthcare Operations Manage-ment*, Chapter 6.)

Checklists

The checklist is one of the seven primary tools of the Six Sigma quality methodology. (The other tools are fishbone diagrams, flowcharts, Pareto charts, histograms, scatter plots, and run charts.) The checklist is a simple

Exhibit 8.3
Patient Check-in
Process Map

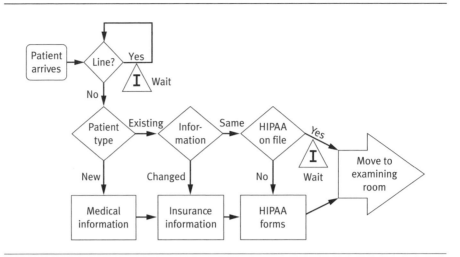

list of the steps in a process, each with a box to check to indicate completion of the task. This relatively simple tool has proven to be powerful and can be easily installed to embed change.

An example of the power of checklists was demonstrated in a study at The Johns Hopkins Hospital on the insertion of central venous catheters. Each year, an estimated 250,000 cases of central line–associated bloodstream infections occur in hospitals in the United States, and an estimated 30,000 to 62,000 of these infected patients die as a result (Gawande 2007). When inserting central line catheters, doctors are supposed to

- wash their hands with soap;
- clean the patient's skin with chlorhexidine antiseptic;
- put sterile drapes over the entire patient;
- wear a sterile mask, hat, gown, and gloves; and
- put a sterile dressing over the catheter site once the line has been inserted.

These steps are accepted practices and have been known and taught for years. However, when the leader of the study (Dr. Peter Pronovost) initially measured their use by ICU doctors, he observed that they skipped one or more steps in more than a third of their patient interactions.

After instituting the use of a checklist for these five steps, Pronovost and his colleagues monitored this procedure for a year. The results were dramatic: The ten-day line-infection rate dropped from 11 percent to zero. Extending the study, they followed their patients for 15 more months. During this period, only two line infections occurred. Assuming the infection rate would not have improved without the checklist, Pronovost and his colleagues concluded that, in this one hospital, use of the checklist presumably prevented 43 infections and eight deaths and saved $2 million in costs.

Control Charts

A key tool that uses balancing feedback to monitor a process is the control chart. The control chart is based on statistical process control (SPC), a statistics-based methodology for determining when a process is veering "out of control." All processes have variation in output; some variation is due to factors that can be identified and managed (*assignable*, or *special*, causes), while other variation is inherent in the process (common causes). SPC is aimed at discovering variation due to assignable causes so that adjustments can be made and "bad" output prevented.

In SPC, measures of a process are taken over time and plotted on a control chart. If the measures follow a normal distribution, only 3 measures out of 1,000 will fall outside +/− 3 standard deviations. The +/− 3 standard deviation limits are the control limits on a control chart.

If a greater number of measures fall outside the control limits (or if the plot follows a statistically unusual pattern), it is likely that the process is experiencing variation due to assignable (i.e., special) causes and is "out of control." The special causes should be found and corrected. After the process is fixed, the measures should fall within the control limits and the process will be, once again, "in control." Exhibit 8.4 is a control chart of inpatient length of stay data generated by SAS statistics software.

Dashboards and Scorecards

The principle of balancing feedback is used more broadly in the *dashboard*. The dashboard concept is based on the automotive dashboard. It provides an easily understood graphical display of key performance data. In many dashboards, actual car gauge symbols are used. Most dashboards display data from multiple databases and in some instances combine the data into graphical displays (see Chapter 3 for examples). Good dashboards have exegetical (drill-down) capability and integrate data from operating systems and data warehouses. Reporting systems are now being deployed that allow managers to create unique dashboards that meet their individual departmental needs.

Exhibit 8.4 Control Chart of Admission Length of Stay Generated with SAS

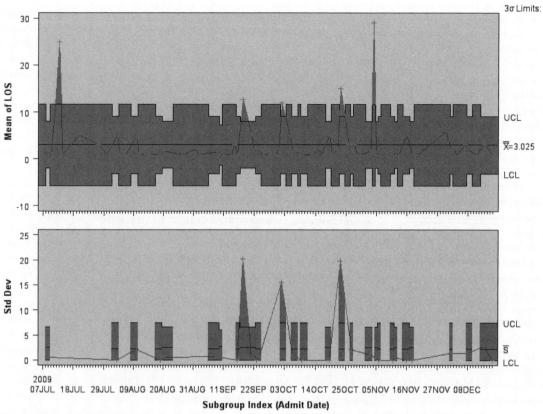

Note that any admission above the Upper Control Limit (UCL) is beyond three standard deviations and "out of control."

Dashboards that include goals are *scorecards*. A common graphical strategy is to place small icons next to scorecard data, in stoplight colors. Green indicates the goals have been met, yellow means the goals have not been fully achieved, and red indicates a problem.

In a study of 109 hospital dashboards, Kroch and colleagues (2006) found three important characteristics of effective dashboards. First, the study indicated that shorter, more focused dashboards that are reviewed on a frequent basis are associated with higher performance. Second, it showed that hospitals with governing boards that more actively use their dashboards for operations management and quality improvement projects are more likely to be high performers. Finally, the study revealed that hospitals perform better when they have highly engaged board quality committees that effectively monitor the quality aspects of the dashboards.

Dashboards and scorecards by themselves are useful. By linking the indicators on the dashboard to the balanced scorecard methodology described in Chapter 5, an even more powerful tool for strategy execution is available to every leader on his or her computer desktop.

Business Rules

The growth of clinical information systems and electronic health records (EHRs) poses a significant opportunity to embed finely tuned clinical and operational systems. However, many healthcare organizations' IT departments are presented with a classic IT dilemma—the software modification queue—as a result of this growth. Because these new systems are complex, changes to the operational systems (e.g., online transaction processing systems) are frequently put in a queue and not delivered in a timely manner.

Just as the personal computer and desktop software (e.g., word processing and spreadsheets) relieved the software modification queue in the 1980s, automated business rules software now accomplishes a similar task—it lets the professional user modify the system to meet his needs. The major difference is that desktop software was intended to be used for local and relatively small data sets. Business rules software, generally called "rules engine" software, is designed to access data warehouses and, in some cases, the operational systems themselves.

Rules engines are used to coordinate a process or apply specialized knowledge. They are usually written in plain English (with some required syntax) and structured with Boolean logic.[1] Each engine contains "terms," which are the data elements (e.g., age, weight, blood pressure), facts (e.g., patient can take medications; the surgery bed 21c is open), and rules (e.g., a man cannot be admitted for childbirth; an account is paid if the balance is zero).

Many organizations outside of healthcare use business rules software extensively. A financial services organization may have a loan application process that contains over 1,000 rules. A major advantage to the use of business rules software is the user's ability to maintain and modify logic without needing help from the IT department. However, along with this freedom comes a responsibility to adequately test and document the procedures that use these rules.

Simple business rules can be implemented with online analytical processing software. For example, a team that is monitoring long stays in the hospital might access its data warehouse to identify patients in need of discharge planning. Exhibit 8.5 shows the data flow in SAS and the filtering rules that create the report shown in Exhibit 8.6 and the Pareto chart shown

Exhibit 8.5 Data Flow and Filtering Rules

Data and report flow

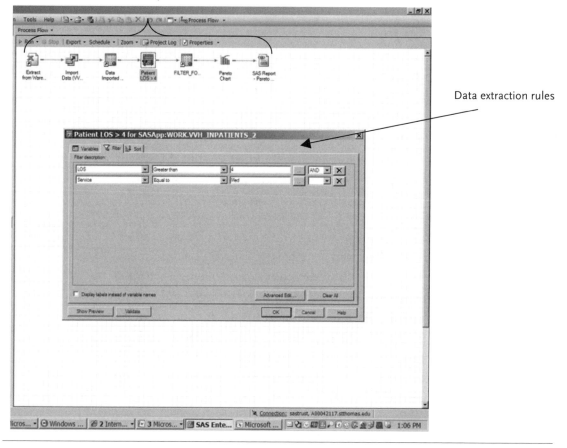

Data extraction rules

in Exhibit 8.7. This rule system can be programmed to run every morning at 8:00 am and to e-mail the results to the discharge planner.

Clinical Decision Support

Most contemporary EHR systems provide some type of clinical decision support, such as drug interaction and patient allergy–drug alerts. However, many vendors are now providing evidence-based software add-ons to these EHR systems that provide care pathways and predetermined disease-specific order sets.

Good clinical support systems prevent clinical complications and help hospitals save money. An evaluation of 167,233 patients at 41 hospitals whose care was rendered using clinical support showed a 21 percent reduction in pneumonia and a 16 percent reduction in patient complications. If extrapolated to the U.S. healthcare system, these improvements could reduce costs

Last	First	LOS	Service
Burrien	Anthony	5	Med
Burrien	Dorothy	6	Med
Duntiels	Glen	5	Med
Ellivan	Gary	8	Med
Flordner	Westin	7	Med
Gutilton	Monty	5	Med
Hankinson	Polly	7	Med
Harpench	Rhonda	11	Med
Jenstiell	Noreg	6	Med
Markina	Danica	8	Med
Mckinner	Lila	8	Med
Monez	Mary	14	Med
Mortes	Terry	8	Med
Nearson	Millie	5	Med
Nearson	Mark	5	Med
News	Jerome	6	Med
Oliamos	Bea	7	Med
Ortinston	Lawrence	9	Med
Schomez	Catherine	8	Med
Stewman	Helma	9	Med
Tershiner	Daniel	5	Med
Vart	Val	8	Med
Warpenez	Everine	6	Med
Wooks	Hila	5	Med
Wooks	Josh	5	Med

**Exhibit 8.6
Length of Stay
Greater than
Four Days Report
Generated Daily
from Data
Warehouse**

by as much as $19 billion per year (Amarasingham et al. 2009). The potential savings per year are even greater in U.S. ambulatory care:

- Preventive care: $1.7 billion to $3.7 billion
- Disease management: $28 billion
- Care of chronic conditions: $139 billion

Together, these savings yield a total cost reduction of between $168.7 billion and $170.7 billion per year.

It is no longer necessary to convene internal experts to develop clinical guidelines, as the federal government, a host of nonprofit quality organizations, and

Exhibit 8.7
Pareto Chart
of Data in
Exhibit 8.6
(sorted by most
frequent
occurrence
of LOS)

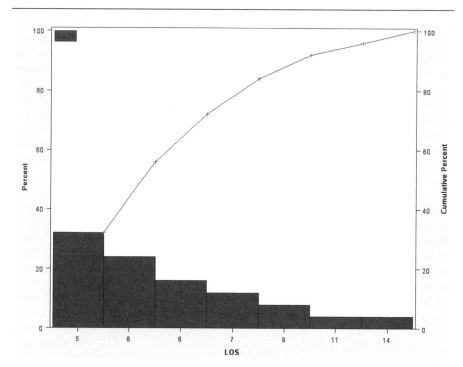

Note the high incidence of LOS = 8, which should be investigated.

software vendors now provide an array of options. The tools and approaches presented in this book provide a system to charter projects to effectively embed these sophisticated clinical decision support tools. In addition, close attention needs to be paid to the user experience to ensure user engagement and effective use of these clinical decision support systems.

Huddles, Transparency, and Face-to-Face Accountability

There are a number of helpful approaches to optimizing the role of people in embedding change. (Section III provides a deeper and broader discussion of the people component of execution.)

A relatively new innovation in healthcare is the *daily huddle*—a short meeting of the staff in a department every day to quickly review the work for the day and identify any problems that need to be addressed. It is helpful to review data and dashboard reports at this meeting as well. Huddles can be used throughout an organization, even at the senior management level. The huddle is an excellent example of providing balancing feedback in a timely manner.

Because of the ubiquitous nature of contemporary computing systems, all employees can access various levels of data. An effective organization shares performance data in a transparent and clear manner. *Transparency* is particularly effective among clinicians, as individuals who are not performing as well as their colleagues can seek advice from them on how to improve. Collegial knowledge transfer is more effective than a directive from a senior manager. In addition, transparency can promote friendly competition among similar departments or units.

Computers may also impede communication—for example, use of e-mail to communicate a sensitive personnel matter may be inappropriate. Regular *face-to-face* communication is one of the salient characteristics of high performing systems. It is important that managers and department directors report their performance and plans for improvement in a periodic face-to-face review meeting with senior management.

NOTES FROM THE FIELD

Vanderbilt Medical Center

The Vanderbilt Medical Center in Nashville, Tennessee, has developed an advanced clinical decision support system that focuses on patient management. Patient management presents many opportunities for error:

- Did the correct drug get ordered?
- Did the nurses provide the therapy on time?
- Did the attending physician respond to the abnormal lab results in a timely manner?
- Did the discharge team know the patient is scheduled to leave today?

In response, Vanderbilt designed a rules engine that works to prevent such problems by including these features:

- Simple rule-based alerts, such as reminders to physicians about possible drug interactions when medications are ordered
- Intelligent synthesis of information about the patient, information from the care setting, and biomedical knowledge (e.g., an antibiotic recommendation based on the patient's condition and a database of the recent sensitivity of microorganisms in the hospital)
- Presentation of information to direct attention to important data (e.g., a dashboard indicating patient status across an entire ward)
- Team-based coordination of care

The Vanderbilt system is "fault tolerant," however. Hospital leaders accept that even the most skilled and committed professional will on occasion provide incomplete or untimely services due to a busy schedule and frequently chaotic environment.

Exhibit 8.8 provides an overview of the Vanderbilt system. Vanderbilt has used this system to reduce the incidence of pneumonia in patients on ventilators. In 2008 Vanderbilt instituted a protocol that included eight procedures that must be delivered to every ventilator patient. It used a specially designed dashboard and alert system to ensure that this protocol was followed every day. The results of using this fault-tolerant system were outstanding. In 2009 the hospital prevented 108 cases of ventilator-associated pneumonia and 16 deaths and saved over $4.3 million in hospital expenses by eliminating 1,066 hospital days that would have been spent treating complications (Schultz 2009). The Vanderbilt system is an excellent example of a combination of clinical knowledge, checklists, and rules engines that provides highly effective reinforcing feedback and supports the delivery of high-quality services consistently over time (Fritz et al. 2010).

SMDC

SMDC (St. Mary's Hospital/Duluth Clinic) bases its performance management approach in its balanced scorecard system of strategy management. Each of the major initiatives on the corporate scorecard is a series of projects that are managed with an adapted IHI style of project management.

A unique feature of the SMDC is the scorecard project reporting icon. For each department (or individual practitioner) there are a number of performance metrics. For those not meeting their goals, the SMDC system requires that a small project plan be attached directly to the scorecard. This attached document is an action plan that will be executed to shift the department's performance results toward the desired goal.

VINCENT VALLEY HEALTHCARE

The VVH medical home team developed a dashboard to track progress on improving preventive services for patients served by this system (see

Exhibit 8.8 Vanderbilt Medical Center Fault-Tolerant Decision Support System

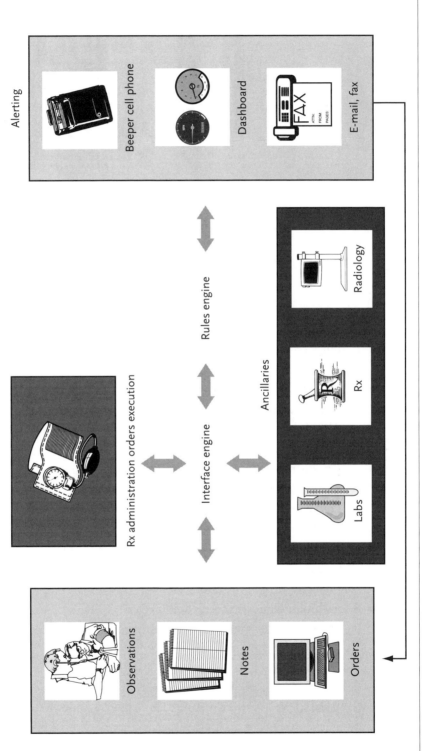

Exhibit 8.9
Medical Home
Preventive
Services
Dashboard

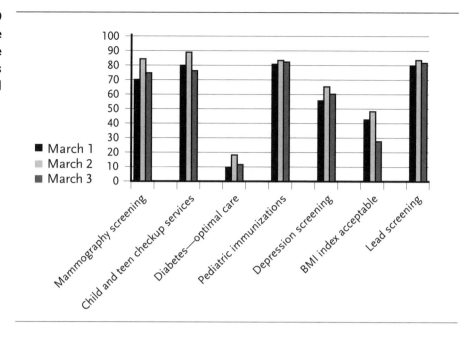

Exhibit 8.9). The numbers in the dashboard represent the percentage of patients receiving the appropriate service or meeting preventive goals in the first three weeks of March.

The VVH ACO team developed a set of business rules to identify patients in need of care management. The rules are run each morning against the VVH data warehouse. Here are the rules:

1. Patient records must be sent to the ACO department if the patient is under management.
2. Patients are under management if they have high use and chronic conditions.
3. High use is charges greater than $1,000 in the last 30 days.
4. Chronic conditions are diabetes, asthma, and congestive heart failure.
5. Diabetes diagnostic codes are: 250.xx.
6. Asthma diagnostic codes are: 493.xx.
7. Congestive heart failure diagnostic codes are: 428.xx.

SUMMARY

Effective strategy execution is critical to high performance healthcare—but almost equally important is embedding changes to ensure processes perform as expected over the long term. Most of the tools that help an organization embed change successfully are based on the General Systems Theory of balancing feedback. Standard operating procedures and process maps document change and help maintain it. Checklists are simple, effective tools that can be used in many clinical environments. Graphic displays of performance through dashboards and scorecards provide timely feedback that is easy to understand.

New computer tools are also being used to embed change. Automated rules engines enable the user to access and process data in a structured manner to monitor and maintain performance. Well-designed clinical decision support systems have been shown to significantly improve the quality and reduce the cost of care. In addition, the use of daily huddles, transparency of data, and structures that foster face-to-face accountability optimize the role of staff in embedding change.

NOTE

1. Boolean logic is named after British mathematician George Boole. It combines propositions with the logical operators AND, OR, IF THEN, EXCEPT, and NOT. The results of these propositions are either TRUE or FALSE.

SECTION III

PEOPLE

You must be the change you wish to see in the world.

Mohandas Gandhi, political and spiritual leader of India

CHAPTER 9

Structure and Compensation

THE STRUCTURE OF an organization can either support or impede its performance. Similarly, the system of employee and physician compensation can also significantly impact the ability of an organization to execute effectively and deliver high-quality results. This chapter provides an overview of contemporary approaches to optimizing structure and compensation systems, including

- fundamentals of effective organizational design,
- new concepts for structuring large organizations,
- effective compensation systems, and
- physician compensation, compacts, and professional services agreements (PSAs).

STATE OF THE ART

Fundamentals of Effective Organizational Design

Poor performance can be a symptom of poor organizational design. Senior management needs to continuously evaluate whether the organization's current structure is executing properly and delivering expected results. Kates and Galbraith (2007) provide a model to be used when considering initial organizational structure or reorganization (see Exhibit 9.1).

As an organization's leaders develop answers to the questions posed by the star model, they have an array of organizational options they can use to meet their strategic goals.

One common option is a *functional organization structure*. A functional structure is useful for a small organization that has a limited scope of business,

**Exhibit 9.1
Star Model of
Organizational
Design**

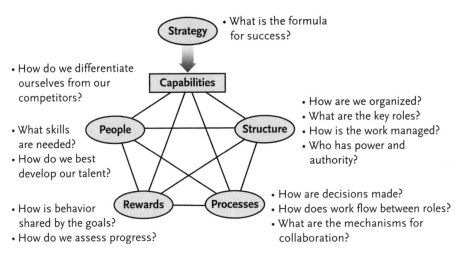

- What is the formula for success?
- How do we differentiate ourselves from our competitors?
- What skills are needed?
- How do we best develop our talent?
- How is behavior shared by the goals?
- How do we assess progress?
- How are we organized?
- What are the key roles?
- How is the work managed?
- Who has power and authority?
- How are decisions made?
- How does work flow between roles?
- What are the mechanisms for collaboration?

Source: Kates and Galbraith, 2007. *Designing Your Organization: Use the Star Model to Solve 5 Critical Design Challenges*. John Wiley & Sons, Inc. Used with permission.

deep expertise in one area, and a relatively stable operating environment. Exhibit 9.2 demonstrates this structure for a small clinic.

The *product structure* is organized around the products or services delivered by the organization. It has these advantages:

- New services can be developed rapidly, because all employees involved in the new product work closely together.
- The focus on one product line fosters innovation and a deep understanding of new products.
- There is a reduced need to coordinate with other parts of the organization to gain approvals for changes because the structure is self-contained.

Exhibit 9.3 is a simplified example of a product structure. Note that the focus of the delivery structure is on the clinical product.

The *customer structure* is built around a common segment of customers/patients. Organizing around customers can be effective, but certain conditions need to be met:

- Staff must have a deep knowledge of this particular type of patient.
- The services provided to each patient segment must be sufficiently unique.
- The volume of services must be large enough to achieve efficiencies of scale.

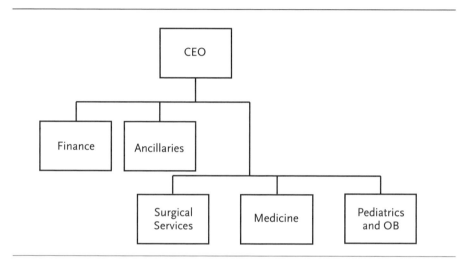

**Exhibit 9.2
Functional
Structure—
Small Clinic**

**Exhibit 9.3
Product
Structure—
Inpatient
Hospital
(simplified)**

An example of an integrated system is shown in Exhibit 9.4. This system is organized around the primary care patient's geographic proximity to the clinic and the level of services needed by the emergency patient.

Many hospitals have vacillated between product structure and customer structure for the organization of inpatient services. For example, some hospitals have combined their cardiac ICU (customer structure) with their general ICU (product structure). Other hospitals have increased the number of general routine beds and eliminated "services" (e.g., medicine, surgery, obstetrics).

All structures create "silos" that prevent people from working together. An effective structural design acknowledges this challenge and uses four tools to overcome it:

- *Networks*: Individuals in an organization create informal relationships with coworkers to coordinate work. Managers can encourage networking by co-locating workers, holding joint meetings and training sessions, rotating work assignments, and using technology to support communications and internal social networking.

**Exhibit 9.4
Customer/
Patient
Structure—
Integrated
System
(simplified)**

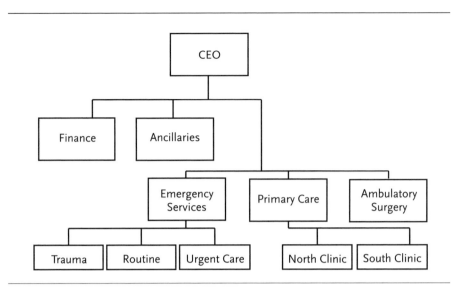

- *Teams*: Teams are individuals brought together to work independently while sharing collective responsibility for outcomes. Teams are more formal than networks and participation is required, not voluntary. All the components of good project management discussed in Chapter 6 apply to teams.
- *Integrative roles*: A full-time manager who orchestrates work across units has an integrative role. This type of manager is accountable for results but does not directly manage the resources needed to achieve the results. An example of this model is the physician–administrator pair (sometimes called a *dyad*), which shares accountability for a clinical service line's performance.
- *Matrix structures*: An employee who reports to two or more parts of an organization is part of a matrix structure. Matrix structures promote flexible and efficient use of resources but must be managed by a sophisticated set of leaders who can deal with the inevitable conflicts this structure fosters.

New Concepts for Structuring Large Organizations

As businesses outside of healthcare have grown, new organizational concepts have emerged. The hierarchical structures of the past had an institutional pyramid structure that emphasized control but were unwieldy and expensive. Smaller, more nimble competitors eventually became more innovative and cost-effective and took market share away from the behemoths.

New structures consider a number of key issues (Roberts 2004):

- *Complementarity*: In the new designs, doing more of one thing increases the returns of another. For example, increasing primary care visits will eventually increase surgeries. However, providing outstanding outpatient care for congestive heart failure will decrease admissions and reduce revenue (hence violates the principle). Organizational design should increase complementarity.
- *Non-concavity and non-convexity*: Many structural designs are improved incrementally (e.g., through a Lean Six Sigma project), but some improvements require discrete, large, structural changes. For example, a new drug may eliminate the need for a surgical procedure—hence performing the surgery slightly more effectively would not be a good strategy. In these non-incremental situations, the organizational designer must operate at a high level (e.g., not with the surgeons) to identify the correct new structure.
- *Cooperation versus initiative*: An organizational unit needs to cooperate with the total firm to achieve strategic objectives. The unit also needs to be creative and show initiative. These two goals sometimes conflict, but they must be encouraged and managed.

  An example is unit-based clinical testing versus the use of a central laboratory. An inpatient hospital unit may decide to purchase a point-of-service blood testing device that provides real-time results to clinicians. This is an example of initiative taken by a unit to speed processes and improve clinical care. However, these blood samples would have normally gone to a centralized lab, where costs are lower and the lab quality control systems are more robust. A good solution to this potential conflict is to have the maintenance and quality assurance of this equipment be overseen by the central lab. Good organizational design fosters both cooperation and initiative.
- *Motivation and performance measures*: Individuals are motivated to perform their jobs by a number of organizational design features. The architect of the structure needs to pay attention to these features as she constructs the metrics for individual performance or team performance. Large modern firms recognize the connection between organizational design and motivation and consider the following principles of structure:
  - Establish clarity about strategy and policies and communicate them effectively
  - Create discrete organizational units that are smaller than the current unit

- Give unit leaders increased operational strategic authority but hold them accountable for results
- Reduce the number of layers of hierarchy
- Reduce the number of central staff positions
- Increase performance incentives at the unit and individual levels
- Increase resources for management training and development and peer knowledge transfer systems

An example of the application of these principals can be seen in the restructuring of a hospital-based ambulatory care department. This department has 300 employees and a management structure that includes 15 managers and their support employees. This unit could be split into five clinics, each having only one manager, all of whom report to a senior executive in the hospital. The five managers would meet as a team and share best practices. The senior executive would set performance metrics and monitor them closely via dashboards (see Chapter 8). This restructuring would eliminate a level of management, and it is more nimble than the original structure.

Effective Compensation Systems

Although the primary reason most individuals work in healthcare is not financial reward, the progressive organization must pay close attention to its compensation systems. It is easy to underestimate the expense and effort necessary to maintain these fundamental characteristics of an effective system:

- Internal equity: Employees doing similar work receive similar pay.
- External equity and competitiveness: The organization is paying enough to attract and retain quality employees (see Chapter 3 on benchmarking).
- Performance monitoring and rewards: Employees understand how their pay will change on the basis of their performance.
- Legalities: All federal and local laws and regulations are followed.

Many organizations have installed variable pay systems based on performance. It is important to design these systems in consideration of the organization's culture. For example, an academic physician's compensation may be only partially based on fees generated because research and teaching are important parts of this job as well. The risk and reward built into these systems need to be carefully constructed so that employees have a realistic opportunity to achieve the goals that will bring them additional compensation.

The most effective variable payment systems are those that have clear metrics. In departments that do not have such metrics, or whose metrics are not sufficiently connected to the department's mission, the manager should be provided a pool of compensation that can be used to adjust each employee's salary individually. Trying to use a compensation system based on quantitative measures in these departments only causes confusion and disappointment.

Physician Compensation, Professional Services Agreements, and Compacts

How to pay doctors is a complex and rapidly changing issue, and this book can provide only guidance on current trends. New compensation systems need to be created because the number of small practices is decreasing and many physicians are choosing to be part of large groups or integrated systems. The major reasons for this shift include financial uncertainty, the need to acquire and maintain electronic health record systems, and lifestyle considerations such as work hours and on-call schedules.

One interesting physician compensation model that helps existing practices deal with these challenges while retaining some measure of autonomy and identity is the *professional services agreement*. Under this arrangement, a health system or hospital employs all the practice's non-physician employees and provides all support services such as billing and electronic health records systems. The providers receive their fee revenue, less a percentage for administrative costs; or they are compensated based on the number of relative value units (RVUs) they produce. The payment per RVU approach removes the risk of a poor payer mix. Although the providers are not under any contractual obligation to refer their patients to the health system (such an obligation would violate federal laws), the PSA promotes a positive relationship that can potentially lead to a closer partnership.

Physician Compacts

A compact is a written agreement between two parties that describes practices that both parties will engage in or refrain from. In the case of physicians, it differs from the more familiar contract in that it has a balanced set of obligations and responsibilities for both the individual and the organization. It is an informal understanding between the physicians and the organization's leadership as to what physicians expect to give to the group and what physicians expect to get from the group in return.

The compact defines the relationship in terms of characteristics that are central to the partnership, such as the support of clinical excellence and financial viability of the organization. It is a social contract, not a legal contract. Compacts can be used during the selection process to communicate to a new physician the organization's values and expectations. In interviews with prospective new providers, compacts also provide an outline that can be used to ascertain candidates' compatibility and fit with the organization. For many organizations, the act of creating the compact is as powerful as the document itself, as it fosters deep discussions on an organization's mission and values.

NOTES FROM THE FIELD

The compact HealthPartners uses for its physicians and dentists is its "Partnership Agreement." This is shown in Exhibit 9.5.

VINCENT VALLEY HEALTHCARE

Structure and the Professional Services Agreement

As Jim Hanson began his work with the clinics in the Tasker Foothills area, he realized that a number of physicians were increasingly tired of the administrative tasks they were required to perform as owners of their practices, such as financial management, personnel matters, and the challenge of selecting and installing health information technology. Many of these same doctors were excited about helping create the medical home model and support its implementation.

Hanson suggested that three of the practices consider a PSA option with VVH, and they agreed. Each clinic maintained its existing name, location, and referral networks. The current support employees were converted to VVH employees, and all financial systems were transferred to VVH. VVH

Exhibit 9.5
HealthPartners
Physician and
Dentist
Partnership
Agreement

Organization Gives

Involve and engage doctors

Involve doctors in strategy, business, and marketing

Include doctors in the development of patient-centered and doctor-efficient practices

Provide opportunities for leadership training

Promote partnership between doctors, staff, and organization

Listen to and be influenced by doctors, assume good intentions, and foster opportunities and forums for doctors to discuss and deliberate important issues

Support a practice that works for both patients and doctors

Be patient centered

Support 6 Aims* practice and remove barriers at the point of care

Provide an environment and tools to ensure satisfying and sustainable practices

Promote trust and accountability within teams and the medical/dental groups

Create opportunities to educate physicians, dentists, and staff about 6 Aims-centered care

Provide support for a healthy and balanced work life for doctors

Respect physicians' and dentists' time to allow care of patients

Grow strong and sustainable clinical practice

Recruit and retain the best people

Market HealthPartners' multispecialty medical and dental groups aggressively

Provide market-based, performance-linked compensation

Acknowledge and reward contributions to patient care and the organization's goals

Create an environment of innovation and learning

Support teaching and research

Demonstrate accessible, accountable, responsive, and empathetic leadership

Understand the complexity of health care delivery and apply best management practices

Seek to understand the clinical perspective

Communicate coherently our mission, vision, direction, and strategy

Help us to understand the complexity of our dynamic business challenges

Provide performance feedback communicated in the spirit of improvement and learning

Recognize the leadership, professionalism, and contributions of doctors

Resolve conflict with openness and empathy

Continued

Exhibit 9.5
Continued
Physician and Dentist Give

Be involved and engaged

Participate in departmental and medical/dental group meetings and activities

Engage and participate in partnership with practice teams, and with clinical and administrative colleagues

Champion processes to improve care systems service and quality

Provide input to strategy, marketing, and operations development

Develop understanding of the business aspects of care delivery

Raise issues and concerns respectfully

Seek to understand the organizational perspective, assume good intent, and collaborate effectively

Demonstrate ownership of your practice and clinic

Excel in clinical expertise and practice

Be patient centered

Pursue clinical practice consistent with the 6 Aims

Advance personal and care team expertise and excellence

Seek and implement best practices of care for patients

Reduce unnecessary variation in care to support quality, reliability, and customized care based on patient needs

Create innovations for care and care delivery and be open to innovations and ideas for improvement needed in our environment

Show flexibility and openness to change

Support our multispecialty group practice

Demonstrate passion and commitment for your practice and our multispecialty medical and dental group

Collaborate within and across disciplines and partners to improve patient care

Promote, refer, and communicate with colleagues effectively

Use resources responsibly and support care delivery systems that improve care and reduce costs effectively

Participate in teaching and research

also financed and installed a new electronic health record system. The financial analysis showed that the clinic physicians in this new structure netted slightly more income than they had previously. In addition, VVH agreed to recruit two new physicians and financially support them for the first two years of their practice.

Exhibit 9.5
Continued

Be a leader

Demonstrate commitment to the organization's mission and vision

Lead as a role model

Support colleagues and partners

Communicate respectfully and thoughtfully

Use a problem-solving approach when identifying issues

Provide leadership to the care team and delegate effectively

Provide recognition and feedback to other doctors and staff

Participate in and support medical/dental group decisions

Seek ways to continually develop leadership and influence skills

* Refers to the "Six Aims for Changing the Health Care System" developed by the Institute for Healthcare Improvement.
Source: HealthPartners, Bloomington, MN. Used with permission.

Variable Compensation

The publicly reported measures for quality were good in these three clinics, but not the best in the area. From his discussions with the clinics' employees, Hanson determined that their documentation could be improved and that the use of patient reminder systems would be valuable. Because the quality measures were clear and public, Hanson felt he could add a variable bonus based on the clinics' performance that would go to the staff—not the physicians. The medical staff agreed with this proposal, and each clinic employee was eligible for a bonus of up to $500 per year based on improvements in these quality scores. After six months, these three clinics were among the top 10 percent in the state for hypertension control, asthma management, and childhood immunizations.

SUMMARY

Organizational performance is affected by organizational design. Organizations need to design structures that are compatible with their strategies, processes, rewards, and employees' skills. Designs may be functional, product oriented, or patient focused. All structures create silos, but their isolating effect can be minimized through the use of networks, teams, integrative roles, and matrix reporting relationships.

New design concepts for large organizations emphasize small unit sizes, significant reduction of all middle layers of management, highly metricized goals and compensation for unit managers, and sharing of best practices among peers.

For an organization to execute effectively, a solid compensation system must be in place to assure and motivate employees. This system must include both internal and external equity. Pay-for-performance systems need to align with organizational strategy, be easily understood by employees, and be considered fair.

Use of the professional services agreement to create new relationships between independent physician practices and larger healthcare organizations has become widespread. Physician compacts can be used to clarify the expected behaviors and relationships between doctors (and other providers) by clearly delineating what each side of the relationship gives and receives.

CHAPTER 10

Culture and Employee Engagement

"It's just how we do things around here." Culture is the unseen force that cements organizations together (or in some cases tears them apart). Culture can be a positive force that drives change and innovation or it can be an overwhelming force that preserves the status quo. Any system for effective execution must be supported by the organization's culture—the best organizations use their culture and effective execution as a key competitive advantage.

This chapter reviews the assumptions and influences that shape organizational culture. In particular, methods of measuring and improving a key element of culture—employee engagement—are detailed. Specifically, the chapter addresses

- the elements of culture,
- the assumptions underlying an organization's culture,
- the shaping and embedding of culture,
- the importance of an engaged workforce,
- the use of engagement surveys, and
- the role of survey analysis in identifying obstacles to engagement.

STATE OF THE ART

The Elements of Culture

There are many ways to view organizational culture, but the model developed by Edgar Schein at the Massachusetts Institute of Technology is a particularly useful construct. Schein (2004, p. 17) defines organizational culture as "a pattern of shared basic assumptions that was learned by a group as it solved its problems of external adaption and internal integration, and has worked well enough to be considered valid, and therefore to be taught to new members as the correct way to perceive, think, and feel in relation to those problems."

Culture is built by an organization's history; if the culture is ineffective, the organization ceases to exist. Because many healthcare organizations have long histories, it is often difficult to trace their cultural roots.

An organization's culture can be thought of as having three levels. The highest and most visible level is where "artifacts" are observed—structures and processes that make the organization operate. "Artifacts include the visible products of a group; its language, its technology and products; its artistic creations; its style as embodied in clothing, manners of address; emotional displays and myths and stories told about the organization; its published lists of values, its observable rituals and ceremonies, and so on" (Schein 2004, p. 25). Below this level are the "espoused beliefs and values," which are embodied in strategies, goals, and mission statements. In most organizations, artifacts are congruent with the espoused beliefs and values.

This model would be easy to understand and implement if it were not for the final level of culture: underlying assumptions—"unconscious, taken for granted beliefs, perceptions, thoughts and feelings" (Schein 2004, p. 26). A visual metaphor is the iceberg (Exhibit 10.1), in which the artifacts and espoused beliefs are visible but the underlying assumptions are massive and deep. For example, an underlying assumption in a public teaching hospital would be that all patients should have the highest level of care regardless of their social status, their income, or whether they have a home.[1] Actions by individual employees that violate the underlying assumptions are not tolerated by the organization.

Cultures are ever evolving in response to external and internal forces. These adaptations reflect the group's ability to cope and learn to reestablish stability, meaning, and predictability. "The culture that eventually evolves . . . is a complex outcome of external pressures, internal potentials, responses to critical events, and, probably to some unknown degree, chance factors that could not be predicted from a knowledge of either the environment or the members" of the group (Schein 2004, p. 134). This evolved culture has changed the underlying assumptions, which in turn affect the espoused values and their artifacts.

Assumptions Underlying an Organization's Culture

Leaders need to understand their organization's culture. Although internal staff can explain it and help them understand it, consultants from outside

Exhibit 10.1
The Iceberg
Metaphor:
Underlying
Assumptions Are
Larger than
Espoused Beliefs

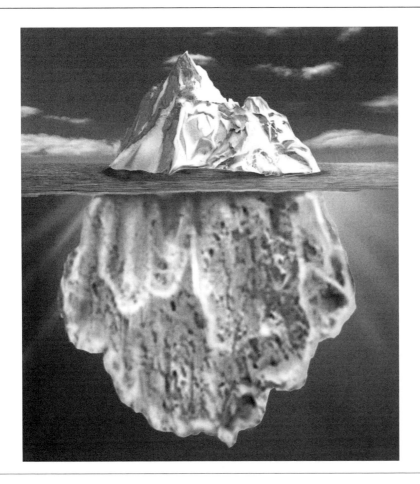

the culture may more easily uncover and communicate the underlying assumptions. The following process can be used to help staff understand an organization's culture:

- Select a facilitator and sample of employees from across the organization.
- Convene a confidential meeting in a safe and comfortable environment.
- Explain the culture model as described earlier.
- Solicit a list of artifacts from the group (e.g., dress codes, layout of work spaces, attitudes, reward structures, requirements for promotion). A useful technique is to ask relatively new employees, "What surprised you about our organization? How is your current job different from your last job(s)?"
- After organizing the artifacts into similar groups, ask participants, "What is going on here? Why are you doing this?" Such questions will help them identify espoused values.

- To uncover underlying assumptions, revisit the artifacts and espoused values to find dissonance. For example, the artifact of publishing quality results online may be supported by the espoused value of "delivery of high-quality care." However if the results that are being reported are lower than expected, the organization should initiate improvement projects. If these projects prove unsuccessful due to lack of physician cooperation, then the underlying assumption of physician autonomy is in conflict with the espoused value of "delivering high-quality care." Successful organizations minimize the dissonance between their espoused values and underlying assumptions.

- After identifying as many underlying assumptions as possible, group them into those that help or hinder organizational performance. Supporting those that help and changing those that hinder are addressed next.

Shaping and Embedding Culture

Leaders can shape cultures; it is perhaps their most important duty. A number of strategies can be used to embed the positive underlying assumptions and change those that hinder organizational progress.

The leader's focus is clearly part of the culture. Because of the transparent reporting tools discussed elsewhere in this book, this leadership focus will be apparent to employees. Also, how the leader reacts in a crisis will indicate which elements of the culture he feels are important. Resource allocations, compensation systems, and promotions also indicate the leader's priorities. For example, the leader who espouses his values by focusing on chronic disease management and population health needs to allocate resources and rewards to primary care clinics, not to highly profitable inpatient services.

The leader's direct relationship with employees also embeds underlying assumptions. It is important for the leader to be a role model, coach, and teacher. Her method of recruiting and the talent she hires and promotes also demonstrate her values and cultural intentions.

Other tools that can be used to embed or change culture include organizational design, key processes design and optimization, physical space design and configurations, ongoing communications about successes and challenges, and formal statements about strategies and values.

The Engaged Workforce

Do your employees look forward to coming to work every day? If they do, you have an engaged workforce. Engaged employees are focused, fully absorbed in their work, and enthusiastic. From an organizational perspective, these employees work proactively, are flexible, are interested in learning new skills, are persistent in the face of obstacles, and readily adapt to change.

Macey and colleagues (2009) describe four factors that are fundamental to an engaged workforce. First, employees must have the *capacity* to engage. They develop this capacity by gaining autonomy and competence. Organizations can support capacity in their employees by sharing information, providing learning opportunities, and encouraging work-life balance.

Employees also need *motivation* to be engaged. Employees are motivated when their work interests them and aligns with their values and they are treated in a manner that reinforces their natural tendency to reciprocate in kind.

Engagement will be low if the work environment is fearful. Therefore, another key factor to successful engagement is *freedom*. Employees need to feel safe to take action on their own initiative—particularly under conditions of adversity, ambiguity, or significant change. Employees must be able to trust the system when they make good-faith efforts to succeed.

Finally, engagement is particularly powerful when it is focused on *strategic alignment*. When employees see a direct connection between what they do and the organization's goals, engagement increases.

Employee Engagement Surveys

Wise organizations continuously evaluate their culture through the use of surveys. The results of periodic surveys are a snapshot of a workforce's engagement and alert managers to problems before they affect organizational performance. An engagement survey also communicates directly to employees the values that senior management has determined are important.

The length of engagement surveys and the frequency with which they are distributed should be carefully considered. The survey must be extensive enough to gather needed information but not so long or frequent that response rates decrease.

Surveys can be created internally or purchased from external vendors. The advantage of using external vendors is that they usually have a number of similar clients and therefore can provide benchmarking data. However, vendor-created surveys are relatively rigid and may not be specific enough to meet an organization's immediate needs.

In addition to survey questions, it is important to craft a transmission message to accompany the survey. This message can include statements such as why the organization feels engagement is important, what an engaged workforce looks like, and what senior management will do with the results.

A comprehensive engagement survey includes questions that address the feelings and behaviors manifested by engaged employees and the four factors that support an engaged workforce: capacity, motivation, freedom, and strategic alignment. Most surveys are made up of positive statements to which employees respond with a Likert scale rating (strongly disagree, disagree, neither agree or disagree, agree, strongly agree).

The following items are examples of statements employees may encounter in an engagement survey (Macey et al. 2009).

Feelings and Behaviors

I feel confident that I can meet my goals.

I am excited about how my work matters to our team and the organization.

Time goes by quickly when I am at work.

Capacity

I have been adequately trained to do my job.

My supervisor sets challenging but achievable goals.

I have enough information to do my job.

I can count on the people I work with to help me if needed.

Motivation

My job makes good use of my skills and abilities.

The people who work here share common values.

The work we do is important.

Freedom

I feel safe to speak my mind about how things can be improved.

I can count on my supervisor to back me up on the actions I take to address a problem.

Strategic Alignment (cost control strategy)

The people I work with maintain their focus on proposing new ways to reduce costs and to be more efficient even when they encounter distractions.

Survey Feedback

After a survey is conducted and the results analyzed and summarized, managers should address any issues they have identified. Senior management is the first to review the results. Benchmarking the results is useful at this stage—both to internal trends and to similar organizations. Statistical analysis can also help senior managers determine which elements of employee engagement are correlated with the structures that support employee capacity building, motivation, freedom, and strategy alignment. Linear regression or similar tools can be used to determine which questions are highly correlated with high or low employee engagement.

The next review occurs at the manager level. The departmental reports should provide enough information that the manager can create an action plan to deal with any areas needing improvement.

Finally, the survey results should be communicated in a summary fashion to the whole organization. This communication should reinforce any themes that were present in the initial communication that accompanied the survey. It should also emphasize the positive aspects of the survey as well as areas that need improvement.

The Agency for Healthcare Research and Quality (AHRQ) has developed an employee engagement survey related to healthcare safety (see www.ahrq.gov/qual/patientsafetyculture). Healthcare organizations may want to select elements of this survey to include in their broader engagement surveys or focus the AHRQ survey on high-risk activities (e.g., surgery suites).

Actions to Improve Engagement

Once engagement issues have been identified in either the organization as a whole or within a single department, leaders can attempt to improve aspects of the work environment affecting engagement. Some suggestions are shown in Exhibit 10.2.

Exhibit 10.2
Interventions
to Improve
Employee
Engagement

Interventions that build confidence and resiliency:
• Provide success experiences for employees
• Provide complete information to employees
• Provide opportunities to learn—and to fail and bounce back
• Provide slack time for updating and training
• Provide performance feedback

Interventions that build social support networks:
• Provide many opportunities (meetings, training, informal gatherings,
  team projects) to facilitate the establishment of social support networks

Interventions that renew or restore employee energy:
• Provide opportunities for balance in employees' lives; do not expect
  continual engagement as engagement can have a "dark side"

Interventions that enhance the motivation to engage:
• Provide jobs that effectively use people's skills
• Provide jobs and a culture that fit employees' values
• Implement effective on-boarding programs
• Provide jobs that permit autonomy of action and choice

Interventions that enhance the freedom to engage:
• Through trust and fairness from:
  – Supervisors
  – "The system"
• Repair trust if the "emotional bank account of trust" has been depleted:
  – Through fair processes
  – Through fair outcomes
  – Through fair interactions with subordinates and coworkers

Leadership as a central intervention in establishing a culture of engagement:
• At all levels
• Especially at the immediate supervisory level

Source: Reprinted from Macey, W. H., B. Schneider, K. M. Barbera, and S. A. Young. 2009.
Employee Engagement: Tools for Analysis, Practice, and Competitive Advantage. Malden, MA:
Wiley Blackwell. Used with permission.

All employees in an organization have an image of the organization's goals, but it is filtered by their job responsibilities, history, and the communications they receive from their managers. Having a clear *line of sight* can significantly improve engagement. When employees have a clear line of sight, they see how their actions help the organization meet its goals (see Exhibit 10.3). "A true line

Exhibit 10.3
Line of Sight

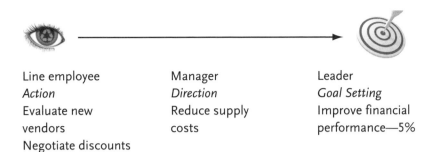

Line employee	Manager	Leader
Action	*Direction*	*Goal Setting*
Evaluate new vendors	Reduce supply costs	Improve financial performance—5%
Negotiate discounts		
Identify new technologies		

of sight is a simplified translation of the business strategy into a language that is relevant to everyone. The essence of that translation is the conversion of favorite words, common terms, and repeated stories into something special and unique in an organization" (Haudan 2008, p. 183).

Line of sight can be improved by discussions between managers and employees regarding how their individual actions affect higher organizational goals. Transparent reporting through the use of scorecards also helps foster discussion on line of sight.

Culture, Engagement, and Leadership

Schein (2004, p. 2) believes that culture and leadership are intrinsically linked: "Leadership is now the ability to step outside the culture that created the leader and to start evolutionary processes that are more adaptive. This ability to perceive the limitations of one's own culture and to evolve the culture adaptively is the essence and ultimate challenge of leadership." Engaged employees allow leaders to build the infrastructure to execute effectively and deliver the highest performance healthcare. The next chapter addresses the challenges of leading in the highly complex world of healthcare.

NOTES FROM THE FIELD

HealthPartners

HealthPartners' culture has been on a transformation journey since Mary Brainerd became CEO. One unusual cultural change strategy was the use of theater. She told this story to the Institute for Healthcare Improvement (2009):

> We had been communicating more to staff about the organizational aspirations, but heard back that they did not understand it. They understood the words, but wanted to know how the organization would be different and how they would know if we were accomplishing the goals.
>
> We used theater to address these concerns by commissioning a play from Mixed Blood Theatre Company. In the play, Fire in the Bones, there is a "before" and "after" theme about what health care is and what it could be. The staff did pre-work before the play, and after each performance we had an open discussion. It was a way we could create dialog and a common experience for our more than 9,000 employees.
>
> This strategy turned out to be a riskier move than I thought! We received a lot of feedback. The good news was that people really felt the "after" scenario connected with the reason they went into health care in the first place. They said things like, "This is the kind of work I wanted to do," "This is what makes health care exciting," and, "This is what my real motivator has always been."
>
> On the other hand, we also heard, "We feel like management and the organizational leadership make decisions without understanding the work we are doing," and, "We feel like we don't have enough involvement in changing the work ourselves." We saw opportunities for change not only from a patient perspective, but also from staff's perspective.
>
> Overall, the play was provocative, so we had real rigorous, emotional discussion afterward, which was not at all easy for us as leadership to hear. But clearly, it was necessary, and we are grateful for the feedback because it will allow us to make sustainable changes.

HealthPartners monitors and maintains its culture through a number of internal employee communication vehicles, including a weekly newsletter/blog that includes many positive stories and kudos for HealthPartners staff. The organization also conducts an annual employee survey (with an 84 percent response rate) and quarterly "pulse" surveys that solicit a sample of employees.

SMDC

SMDC also conducts an annual employee engagement survey. This survey, called the "Vital Signs" survey, includes 21 questions. The results are reported to the board and senior leadership and are part of each manager's performance review. The senior vice president for human resources also maintains a daily blog, generates newsletters, and sends e-mail blasts on current urgent issues.

Culture management at SMDC is embodied in transparency and accountability. Through the use of balanced scorecard and dashboard reporting, all managers understand their goals and those of their colleagues. In addition, individual and departmental progress and challenges are widely shared to encourage collegial support and problem solving.

A key cultural challenge is the behavior of senior management in a crisis. In 2009, almost all healthcare organizations faced financial pressures, and some made radical cuts. SMDC was ahead of the curve; senior staff had closely observed their own data that indicated a slowing of the healthcare economy as early as January 2008. They undertook a hiring review process that carefully reduced staff by 200 full-time equivalents over the subsequent 18 months. SMDC leaders also intensely reviewed their strategy maps, metrics, and organizational strengths and decided that no further changes were needed.

The leaders' decision to remain steadfast strongly communicated that the system of transparency and accountability was working and would remain an important part of SMDC's culture in the future.

VINCENT VALLEY HEALTHCARE

Culture Analysis—ACE Project

Phyllis Colson, the manager of the surgical arm of the ACE project, was concerned that the culture of the VVH surgical service might need to change to successfully execute this new bundled payment project. She worked with the VVH organizational development staff to identify a consultant who could help her understand the service's culture and suggest actions to improve areas that would impede this project. The consultant, Julie Hammond, convened an off-site retreat and evaluated the culture as described earlier in the chapter. In addition, Hammond recommended actions Colson could take to improve the surgical services culture. Four significant underlying assumptions, based on observed artifacts and, in some cases, espoused values, were discovered (see Exhibit 10.4).

Exhibit 10.4
Cultural
Assumptions
Underlying
VVH Surgical
Services

Artifacts	Espoused Value	Underlying Assumption
• Poor results shown on scorecards do not lead to consequences. • When discussing data, surgeons routinely open conversations with "those data must be wrong."	We are science-based providers.	Data from management are always wrong.
• All referrals stay inside VVH even when a more appropriate outside provider should be used. • Communications to outside providers are not timely.	We provide the highest quality care.	Outside providers deliver poor care.
• The lead surgeons have aggressively installed clinical decision support systems into the VVH EHR. • Publicly reported quality indicators are in the top 25% in the state.	We provide the highest quality care.	We believe in evidence-based medicine.
• The surgeons use "shared decision making" when discussing surgical options with patients. • Patients are part of process-redesign projects.	We deliver patient-centered care.	Patients need to be part of the care process.

Hammond suggested that the first two underlying assumption be changed and the last two be reinforced. She recommended the following actions:

- Colson will convene a meeting with Bob Olson (COO), Aaron Martin (CIO), and Dr. Terry McCollum (chief of orthopedics) to discuss data issues. Whenever data are questioned, the VVH IT department will provide an audit trail and, if errors are found, make permanent system corrections.
- Colson will organize an evening reception and meeting for key VVH surgical service staff and all the outside providers who will play key roles in the ACE project. During this meeting, the outside providers will present their services in a comprehensive manner, and they and VVH staff will present scientific papers and best practices. Such receptions will be held once every other month.
- Dr. McCollum and Colson will continue encouraging, measuring, and celebrating the use of evidence-based medicine and patient engagement in the surgical services.

Employee Engagement—Medical Home

Jim Hanson felt it was important to measure the engagement level of all employees in the Foothills practices who would be part of the medical home project. He created a simple survey (Exhibit 10.5).

SUMMARY

Organizations that execute effectively pay close attention to their culture and promote engagement in their workforce. Culture is a pattern of shared assumptions that is taught to new employees as the correct way to think, feel, and act in performing their work.

Culture has three levels—the artifacts or behaviors that are visible to all, espoused values that are frequently cited by leaders and managers, and underlying assumptions that drive both espoused values and artifacts. Once an organization discovers its underlying assumptions, it can reinforce the positive assumptions and change those that hinder organizational performance. One key driver of culture is leaders' activities: where they focus, how they respond to crises, and how they select and nurture new employees and handle other personnel actions.

Exhibit 10.5
Employee
Engagement
Survey

I feel confident that I can meet my goals.	SA	A	N	D	SD
Time goes by quickly when I am at work.	SA	A	N	D	SD
I know what is expected of me.	SA	A	N	D	SD
I have the materials, data, and equipment to do my work.	SA	A	N	D	SD
The work we do is important.	SA	A	N	D	SD
I feel safe to speak my mind about how things can be improved.	SA	A	N	D	SD
I have been praised or received recognition in the last month.	SA	A	N	D	SD
I have the opportunity to learn and grow.	SA	A	N	D	SD
I feel a part of the mission of our practice.	SA	A	N	D	SD

Comments:

_____

_____

_____

_____

SA = strongly agree, A = agree, N = neutral, D = disagree, SD = strongly disagree

Closely related to culture is employee engagement. Engaged employees drive performance, innovation, and change. Four factors influence engagement: the capacity to engage, motivation for engagement, freedom to take action without fear of retribution, and alignment of work with organizational goals. Employee surveys are useful for monitoring engagement.

Culture and employee engagement are the foundations necessary for successful implementation of the leadership approaches presented in Chapter 11.

NOTE

1. The author was the CEO of a public teaching hospital and observed a number of employee incidents that violated this underlying assumption. These employees were made to feel unwelcome by their coworkers after these incidents and resigned soon thereafter.

Leadership

THE FIRST TWO sections of this book provided systems for creating and executing strategic plans. However, neither of these activities is effective without strong leadership, an engaged workforce, and a structure and compensation system to support this work. In contrast to the business tools rooted in mathematics and engineering outlined in sections I and II, the people skills discussed in Section III are based on many years of research and application in the fields of psychology and sociology.

This chapter focuses on individual leadership and is based on over ten years of leadership training experienced by practicing physicians and healthcare executives at the University of St. Thomas. Major topics include

- technical versus adaptive work,
- the danger of leadership,
- tools for successfully executing adaptive change,
- servant leadership,
- the physician as leader, and
- the IHI leadership model.

This chapter does not include a "Notes from the Field" section. Instead, this chapter concludes with two extensive VVH examples. These examples are an amalgam of the many cases and leadership successes experienced by participants in the University of St. Thomas' Physician Leadership College and other related professional development programs.

STATE OF THE ART

Adaptive Leadership

There are many leadership theories, consultants, and books available to the healthcare manager today. Many are based on the "great man" theory of leadership, which attributes the success of an organization to an individual's personality and drive. However, the great man approach is not useful to a manager who seeks to adopt behaviors that enable him to lead more effectively.

A more practical and systematic approach to leadership has been developed by Ron Heifetz and Marty Linsky (2002) at Harvard. Their approach, known as Adaptive Leadership, is based on extensive research on human behavior.

Technical Versus Adaptive Work
The first key concept in Adaptive Leadership is that there is a difference between technical and adaptive work. Technical work uses existing knowledge and skills to solve problems, while adaptive work requires a group or team to generate new knowledge, skills, and behaviors. For example, let's assume a clinic has a spike in patient visits. Adding computer workstations to meet this demand would be technical work. Changing the way the data in the system are used to treat patients would be adaptive work.

A fundamental problem occurs when leaders confuse technical and adaptive challenges. Applying a technical fix to an adaptive problem does not institute long-lasting change and may hurt the individuals affected by the change. Such fixes are often applied in healthcare because many clinical and operational issues are technical in nature and physicians and other professional staff have been trained as scientists.

Adaptive problems cannot be solved successfully by a leader who provides answers based solely on the authority structures and without intensive engagement with those actually doing the work. Adaptive work creates and demands independence and interdependence.

From a practical perspective, a mix of adaptive and technical work is needed to surmount almost all execution challenges. The wise leader understands the difference and leads accordingly.

Danger of Leadership
Leadership is a dangerous endeavor. Ask any leader who has attempted a significant adaptive change and you will hear phrases like "I felt I was on a high wire," I didn't know whom to trust," or "I did not believe we would survive the changes."

One basic reason leadership is dangerous is that organizations try to find a way to restore equilibrium when someone upsets the balance. Organizations want to protect themselves from the pain of doing adaptive work; therefore, the leader is frequently at risk.

When a leader initiates an adaptive change, the negative responses can take several forms. The leader can be marginalized by having her authority diminished or even given to someone else. A leader can be diverted from her primary tasks—she can be given a broadened agenda or more responsibilities, or she can be moved to other projects that have "higher priority." The leader can be subjected to personal attack, which can turn the attention away from the adaptive change and onto the character and style of the leader. Another possibility is seduction—the leader may be given an opportunity to lead a more interesting or prestigious project, which compels her to abandon her current difficult adaptive challenge.

While it does not completely eliminate these dangers, the Adaptive Leadership approach described next minimizes them.

Tools for Executing Adaptive Change Successfully
Heifetz identifies four key tools for implementing needed changes.

Get on the Balcony   The first step is to accurately see the situation as it is occurring. The metaphor is "Get on the balcony," meaning the leader must simultaneously participate in a meeting and observe the behavior of the participants—including himself. For example, the leader of an IT team could participate in a meeting and make these observations:

- Everyone on the team seems distracted and under pressure.
- Dr. Smith seems to be particularly angry about the proposed changes.
- No one can keep to the subject.
- The leader's boss is supportive.
- Bill Anderson is dominating the conversation.

If the IT director was not "on the balcony" he might exit the meeting with quite different impressions:

- That was a waste of time.
- We are not sure what we are doing next.
- I need to get back to my real job.

Trying to ascertain "where people are at" requires artful listening skills. Heifetz describes this skill as "listening to the song beneath the words." For example, the reason Dr. Smith may be angry is that his colleagues are criticizing him for not representing them well in this committee. Therefore, he feels the need to be aggressive even though he may agree with the general direction of the team.

Self-reflection by a leader does not occur naturally. It is important for a leader to get past his blind spots. Only then can he begin to understand the emotions of team members, which is vital to securing their support for the adaptive change.

A simple practice for a leader is to take ten minutes after a meeting for quiet reflection and note taking on each team member's behaviors, attitudes, participation, and position on issues. During this reflection, the leader can try to figure out the social systems and interactions that were present in the meeting and determine how well he fit into this system or conflicted with it.

Think Politically   The term *politics* usually has a negative connotation in the organizational environment. However, most successful adaptive change requires the leader to employ skills used by the best (and most ethical) politicians.

An essential element of this political skill is to develop a broad network. This network can be used to find and engage partners who support the change. The network also will identify opponents to the change; it is important to keep these individuals engaged in the discussions and change activities. Although they may disagree with the change, they will appreciate being included and treated respectfully.

Because adaptive change usually involves many individuals, the leader needs to "take the helm" and personally direct the change. He must also acknowledge that change is painful for many individuals and that he appreciates their sacrifices.

Finally, sometimes change is so powerful that some individuals cannot accept it. There may be casualties during an adaptive change, and the leader and the organization must acknowledge this reality.

Orchestrate the Conflict   Because conflict is almost a certainty in major adaptive change, the skilled leader learns to orchestrate it.

The first tactic is to create a "holding environment." This place can be an off-site meeting area; the key element of the environment is that it is a place where people feel that they are safe and can trust others. "In a holding environment, with structural, procedural, or virtual boundaries, people feel safe enough to address problems that are difficult, not only because they strain ingenuity, but because they strain relationships" (Heifetz and Linsky 2002, p. 103).

Team discussions can be led by the team leader or an outside facilitator. The discussion needs to use a shared language, acknowledge the organization's history, and have a clear set of rules. In the holding environment, ideas are more important than hierarchy.

In the discussions in the holding environment, the leader needs to be attuned to the team's engagement and feelings (by being "on the balcony"). The leader must "control the temperature" of the discussion. She can heat it up by asking tough questions, giving people more responsibility than they are comfortable with, exposing conflicts, and protecting the gadflies and oddballs in the group. She can also turn the heat down by addressing technical issues or establishing procedures to solve problems. Or the leader can temporarily reclaim an issue for herself by saying "Let me work on this myself and I will bring my thoughts back to the group." Throughout these discussions it is important for the leader to continuously show team members the future they are striving to achieve.

Only by controlling the temperature of the discussion and pacing the work can true adaptive change be made. With too hot and fast a discussion a project can implode in acrimony. Too low a temperature and pace will not achieve the desired results.

Another important aspect of orchestrating the conflict is to *give the work back* to the team. Long-lasting change is best accomplished by the team, not the leader. This transfer is hard for a manager who prides herself on being a problem solver. She should not remove herself from the work completely but intervene when needed by making observations, asking questions, offering interpretations, and taking action when necessary.

Hold Steady   The final tool the leader needs to successfully make adaptive change is the ability to hold steady and keep focused on the goal. One of the key barriers to effective execution in healthcare is leaders' inability to persist in a rapidly changing environment.

Holding steady also means the leader needs to take the heat for all the tasks that are part of the change. Some of these tasks may need to "ripen" (become acceptable to the group) before they can be implemented, but the leader needs to hold steady to ensure their implementation.

Servant Leadership

Servant leadership, a concept developed by Robert Greenleaf in 1970, is a useful approach to leading in a healthcare environment. Greenleaf distinguishes the servant leader from the power leader. The servant leader lives the *service first* model of leadership, while the power leader uses the *leader first* model (Keith 2001).

Although it is still widely used, there are significant problems with the power leader approach. Power leaders tend to focus on having power, not on using it wisely. The leader's measure of success is gaining more power for himself, not improving the organization. This focus promotes conflict and internal politics as subordinates strive to be on the winning side. This internal conflict may mask organizational issues that need to be solved and may cause the organization to miss opportunities in external markets.

In contrast, servant leaders use power to serve the organization, not themselves. The classic servant leader was George Washington. After leading the Revolutionary War and serving two terms as president, he stepped down and returned to farming. He was so popular he could have become the "King of America" but instead chose to serve the broader needs of a new nation by stepping down and allowing for an orderly change of power.

Servant leaders today demonstrate seven key practices:

1. *Self-awareness*. Servant leaders are fully aware of their strengths and weaknesses. As a result, they are less likely to judge and more likely to encourage their colleagues. They appreciate teams for the mix of skills members contribute. Self-awareness is closely connected to "getting on the balcony" as described by Heifetz.

2. *Listening*. It is difficult for highly educated and talented leaders to listen, as they frequently feel they see the answer immediately. The servant leader trains himself to be a disciplined listener. "They listen to individuals face to face. They observe what people are doing. They ask questions. They conduct informal interviews, formal interviews, surveys, discussion groups, and focus groups. They use suggestion boxes. They are always listening, watching, and thinking about what they can learn" (Keith 2001, p. 37).

3. *Changing the pyramid*. Instead of sitting at the top of a hierarchical structure, servant leaders work in teams where the team leader is *primus inter pares*, or "first among equals." This approach is particularly effective in healthcare, where a strong sense of professionalism and collegiality are part of most successful cultures. In addition, this approach focuses on meeting patients' needs as opposed to those of the boss.

4. *Developing colleagues*. Every leader has colleagues with whom he works closely. The servant leader seeks ways to support his colleagues' work and success. He also collaborates with colleagues on new initiatives that can promote professional development for all.

5. *Coaching, not controlling.* Although most leaders have subordinates, the servant leader approaches this relationship from the perspective of coaching, not directing. The servant leader believes that "people do their best when they are taught, mentored, and coached, benefitting from both positive and negative feedback as they make their daily decisions and do their daily work" (Keith 2001, p. 46).

6. *Unleashing the intelligence and energy of others.* Servant leaders believe in empowerment. *Empowerment* means involving the people who are doing the work in decisions that affect their roles and goals or, as Heifetz would say, giving the work back to the people.

7. *Foresight.* Leaders have a responsibility to not only develop specific strategic plans but also continuously evaluate how the past and present connect to the future. The six preceding practices are important in developing this capability, as is the use of scenarios to explore possible futures (see Chapter 4).

Physician Leadership

As healthcare systems execute new systems of care in response to healthcare reform, physician leadership is critical. A recent study by McKinsey & Company "found that hospitals with the greatest clinician participation in management scored about 50 percent higher on important drivers of performance than hospitals with low levels of clinical leadership did" (Mountford and Webb 2009). The Adaptive Leadership and servant leadership models just described are key concepts in developing physician leaders.

However, many physicians are reluctant to take on leadership roles. Some are reluctant to take on vague leadership responsibilities (and related people issues) when they are accustomed to the immediate values and rewards of patient care. The career path for physician leaders is frequently unclear, and in some organizations, physicians in leadership positions earn less than clinicians. Training for these roles is usually minimal, and some doctors who have spent years learning clinical skills are concerned that they do not have the academic underpinnings to be effective leaders and managers. Finally, leadership is a lonely job.

Many physicians do become effective leaders, predominantly due to the support their organizations provide. This support includes disciplined cultural change (see Chapter 10) that celebrates and rewards physician leaders' achievements. In these organizations, disincentives to leadership by physicians—such as inadequate compensation, time, and support staff—are eliminated. Finally, lifelong learning for leadership skills is supported and funded either within the organization or in partnership with external resources.

The focus of these educational activities has been summarized by Dr. James Stoller (2008) of the Cleveland Clinic. He extensively reviewed the physician leadership literature and identified six domains of skills needed by physician leaders. They include:

1. Technical knowledge and skills (e.g., of operations, finance and accounting, information technology and systems, human resources [including diversity], strategic planning, legal issues in healthcare, and public policy)
2. Knowledge of healthcare (e.g., of reimbursement strategies, legislation and regulation, quality assessment, and management)
3. Problem-solving prowess (e.g., regarding organizational strategy and project management)
4. Emotional intelligence (e.g., the ability to evaluate self and others and to manage oneself in the context of a group)
5. Communication (e.g., in leading change in groups and in individual encounters, such as in negotiation and conflict resolution)
6. A commitment to lifelong learning

The IHI Model

The Institute for Healthcare Improvement supports many clinical quality improvement efforts both in the United States and internationally. IHI has developed a leadership framework whose core is: will, ideas, and execution.

"In order to get organization-level results, leaders must develop the organizational *will* to achieve them, generate or find strong enough *ideas* for improvement, and then *execute* those ideas—make real improvements, spread those improvements across all areas that would benefit, and sustain the improvement over time. And when this Will-Ideas-Execution framework is fully fleshed out with the addition of two other core components, 'Set Direction' and 'Establish the Foundation,' 24 specific elements emerge into an overall leadership system for improvement called the IHI Framework for Leadership for Improvement" (Exhibit 11.1) (Reinertsen, Bisognano, and Pugh 2008).

The IHI framework includes many of the tools contained in sections I and II. The "Execute Change" step can be led using both the adaptive and servant leadership models.

Exhibit 11.1 IHI Framework for Leadership for Improvement

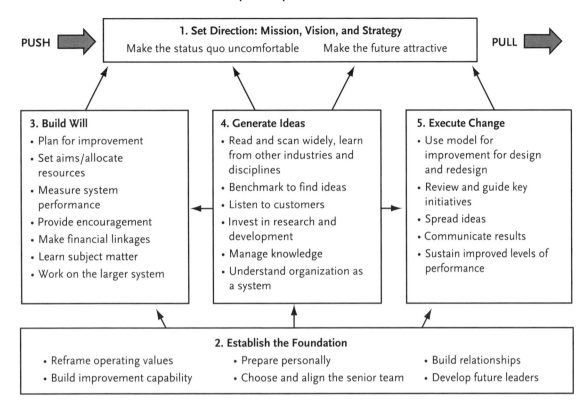

Source: Reinertsen JL, Bisognano M, and Pugh MD. *Seven Leadership Leverage Points for Organization-Level Improvement in Health Care* (Second Edition). IHI Innovation Series white paper. Cambridge, MA: Institute for Healthcare Improvement, 2008. (Available on www.IHI.org.) Used with permission.

VINCENT VALLEY HEALTHCARE

Adaptive Leadership and the ACO Project

Sally Campion realized soon after taking on the accountable care organization (ACO) project that most VVH staff felt the project was just a new financing vehicle and that it primarily affected the hospital's payment systems and electronic health record (EHR). Campion knew that her staff could make some contributions to care management for ACO enrollees who had chronic diseases but that many other individuals—particularly the primary care physicians—needed to change their approach to the management of their patients.

Dr. Robert Munsey is the chief of family medicine at VVH. He has 25 staff physicians and a medical residency program with 20 residents. Their clinics were busy—especially with a recent influx of non-English-speaking

Technical change

Adaptive change

patients. Dr. Munsey was somewhat irritated that the ACO project did not include his department and, therefore, was not inclined to be helpful.

Campion's ACO staff were reporting poor responses from the family medicine staff when patient management issues were brought to their attention even though everyone had agreed to evidence-based guidelines at the outset of the ACO project. Campion felt she would be unable to effect change in the family medicine department and asked Dr. Ira Moscone (CMO of VVH) for help.

Creating a holding environment

Dr. Moscone decided to convene the medical leadership from pediatrics, family medicine, and internal medicine and the ACO staff to see if they could improve the functioning of the ACO team. He rented a conference space at a pleasant retreat center approximately 60 miles west of VVH.

Thinking politically

Everyone agreed to spend a whole day there (with cell phones off). Before the meeting, Dr. Moscone went out of his way to talk to as many physicians as he could in the three departments to understand their concerns about the ACO project and their suggestions for it. During these conversations,

Danger—diversion to projects with perceived higher priority

he learned that some physicians were questioning his involvement in the ACO project; they thought he should be focusing on helping CEO Susan Francis resolve the governance challenges for VVH.

Getting on the balcony

At the beginning of the meeting at the retreat center, Dr. Moscone asked Campion to provide an overview of the ACO project, its current status, and issues she was encountering. After this presentation, Dr. Munsey provided his perspective that only primary care physicians, especially family medicine doctors, should manage patients with chronic diseases. How could a team of nurses and care managers in a different building manage these complex patients? (Dr. Moscone understood that the "song beneath the words" was Dr. Munsey's long-standing concern that his doctors were not respected by the rest of the VVH medical staff. Most of the staff expansion and capital expenditures had been directed to other medical specialties over the previous decade. By assigning these tasks to nurses, VVH was once again disrespecting family medicine.) In response, Dr. Moscone stated that the success of the ACO project depended on the expertise and experience of the primary care physicians at VVH. In addition, this project was highly visible inside VVH, and its success would be an important validation of all of the good work done by these departments over many years.

Turning up the heat

Dr. Moscone next asked all of the members of the group—both physicians and nurses—to explain how they thought the system should work, particularly the interface between the ACO nurses and the physicians. After each nurse presented her thoughts, Dr. Moscone asked the three physician leaders why the system wasn't working, what could be done about it, and how soon. Dr. Maria Sanchez, chief of pediatrics, said that the VVH EHR system did not indicate if her patients were in the ACO project or if any of the special procedures the team had developed for care management should be used. Dr. Moscone said her observation was important and that he would ask CIO Aaron Martin to make this change to the system a high priority. As they broke for lunch, Dr. Moscone felt comfortable that the group was making progress and starting to work well together. He broke the group into four small teams after lunch and asked them to devise solutions to a number of the operating issues that Campion had addressed initially. They were instructed to bring back their solutions at the end of the day.

Turning down the heat by addressing technical issues

Giving the work back to the people

Holding steady

At the end of the meeting, all of the participants agreed that much progress had been made. The ACO staff would develop a scorecard with metrics for this project and make it available throughout VVH. They also agreed to meet quarterly in this type of environment to work out any other problems that might arise as the project matured.

Servant Leadership and the Medical Home Project

Dr. Cynthia Andresen had participated in the decision to hire Jim Hanson as the project manager for the Tasker Foothills medical home project. They spent the first few weeks working on a detailed project plan, but they soon realized that many of the tasks and the schedule were dependent on how well the other practices in the Foothills area came on board and engaged.

Dr. Andresen was respected by her colleagues in the area, but she realized that her personality was not well suited to a highly visible and aggressive leadership style. However, she did like helping others succeed, so she and Hanson agreed that she could easily use a servant leadership approach to this project. The first step was to schedule appointments with the physician leaders of the other Foothills practices involved in the project to hear their perspectives. She was careful during these meetings to gather input and ideas and avoided trying to sell the project.

Self-awareness

Listening

The next step was the creation of an academic journal club for doctors in the area. The club met biweekly for dinner, and members listened to one doctor present an interesting recent journal article. Dr. Andresen acted as the host for these events and the lively discussion that always ensued. These meetings built trust and collegiality, which was essential for implementing the medical home project.

Developing your colleagues

Once a number of the practices in the area had committed to the project, they decided some sort of loose governance would be useful. Dr. Andresen created an advisory board for the project and served as its first chair. However, she made it clear that she would serve in the role for only two years. Thereafter, another physician leader could be elected.

Changing the pyramid

Unleashing the
intelligence and
energy of others

Coaching, not
controlling

Foresight

On the basis of the advisory board's input, Hanson worked with the VVH training department to create professional development classes for the staff of each of the clinics. The department also helped some physicians learn coaching skills to enable them to deal with some challenging but talented employees.

Finally, Dr. Andresen and Hanson used the Learning School planning approach with the Advisory Committee to construct and update a strategic plan for the clinics. Because of the trust the Advisory Committee had in Hanson's skills, the amount of physician time needed to establish this plan and ensure its effective execution was minimal.

SUMMARY

Effective execution begins and ends with effective leadership. The Adaptive Leadership model is particularly useful for healthcare organizations, as it separates technical change from adaptive change. Adaptive change requires a group or team to generate and use new knowledge, skills, and behaviors. Leading adaptive change is dangerous. The Adaptive Leadership approach provides four tools the leader can use to surmount the danger and successfully lead the change:

- "Get on the balcony" and understand the dynamics and social structure of the change
- Think politically and develop a network of supporters
- Orchestrate the conflict that will naturally occur by controlling the heat of the discussion and the rapidity of change
- Hold steady to ensure that the change will occur and be embedded

Another useful approach for healthcare leaders is to become a servant leader. These leaders demonstrate self-awareness, listening skills, and a nonhierarchical style and coach and develop their colleagues and direct reports to unleash their skills and energy.

The need for physician leaders is increasing; many of the most effective healthcare organizations today are physician led. Physicians in leadership positions should be supported through appropriate compensation, support staff, requisite authority, and ongoing training in leadership and business skills.

SECTION IV

AN INTEGRATED SYSTEM

You give an order around here and if you can figure out what happens to it after that, you're a better person than I am.

Harry S. Truman, 33rd president of the United States

CHAPTER 12

An Integrated System
for Execution

EVEN THE PRESIDENT of the United States can find that implementing his plans is difficult; the challenge of execution is pervasive. However, the tools and people skills outlined in this book can be used to form an integrated system to effectively execute strategy and achieve high performance healthcare.

This final chapter provides a path to the future and reviews these concepts:

- How strategy formulation, business tools, and people skills form an integrated system
- Chaos and the unexpected
- The Baldrige Award
- An action plan for improvement of an organization's execution skills

STATE OF THE ART

The Integrated System

Effective execution is based on systems thinking, data-driven decision making, and respect and support for an organization's people. A systems view of this execution methodology is illustrated in Exhibit 12.1. Every organization has data and people, which are the foundations for execution. For effective execution to occur these assets must be integrated with the business tools of strategy development, project management, and embedding systems. These tools must be implemented in a manner that allows real-time sensing and change control based on data. The data must be maintained in accurate and timely warehouses with user-friendly analytics tools.

Exhibit 12.1
An Integrated
System for
Execution

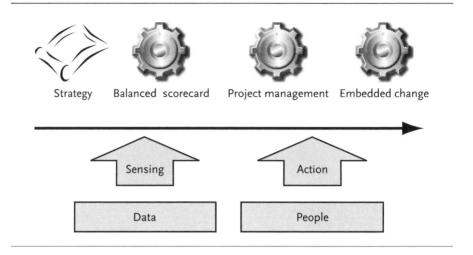

In addition, these tools rely on a support structure that empowers an organization's people. People must be organized and compensated in systems that encourage performance. Finally, an organization's culture and leadership methods are, in the end, the most important elements of the strategy execution system.

Chaos and the Unexpected

Some might criticize this integrated approach to execution as too cumbersome to respond to unexpected events, or they may suggest it would not work in an organizational environment that is chaotic. Many physicians today feel that they practice in chaotic environments due to the pressure of new technologies, changing payer requirements, new professional relationships, Internet-empowered patients, and many other factors. They map this chaotic outlook onto any organizational structure in which they reside, making planning and execution difficult.

However, the execution system outlined in this book is based on systems theory and is highly robust in times of rapid or unexpected change. The development of strategic plans can proceed in a number of ways; the Learning School approach is particularly flexible when leaders are confronted with an unexpected challenge or opportunity. Scenario planning also helps leaders anticipate change and develop dynamic strategies to succeed in a variety of environments.

The business tools in this integrated system are all data based and provide timely feedback on the execution of strategies and overall organizational performance. Organizations that effectively use these tools are not taken by surprise when a department or an individual practitioner does not perform well, and can take steps quickly to ameliorate any negative impact. Organizations that pay attention to their structure, compensation, culture, and leadership approach understand how to use these assets to surmount challenges and avoid chaos.

Assume Medicare makes a payment policy decision that was unexpected and would severely impact the revenue generated by an organization's cardiologists. A well-executing organization would quickly review its strategic plan and strategy maps to establish a new initiative on cardiology revenue. It would charter a project team that included individuals who are trained in project management, understand the culture, and have both adaptive and servant leadership skills. The team would carefully analyze existing data and develop new approaches to generating cardiology revenue or reducing costs. Scorecards would be implemented to measure success, and decision-support rules would be added to the organization's EHR. A cardiologist who was part of this organization could take comfort that appropriate and effective solutions would be developed that would maintain a stable and supportive environment for her practice.

The Baldrige Award

Since 2002, the U.S. Department of Commerce has awarded a special Malcolm Baldrige Award for performance excellence in healthcare (Baldrige National Quality Program 2010). Healthcare organizations applying for this award must demonstrate high performance in the following categories:

1. Leadership
2. Strategic planning
3. Customer focus
4. Measurement, analysis, and knowledge management
5. Workforce focus
6. Process management
7. Results

John Griffith, a professor of health administration at the University of Michigan, reviewed the ongoing performance of winners of the award since 2005 (Griffith 2009). The results were stunning. Baldrige Award winners showed continuing top performance in quality benchmarks, patient and customer satisfaction, financial stability, worker satisfaction and retention, physician satisfaction, and efficiency and cost control. In many of these categories, the hospitals' performance ranked in the top 10 percent of healthcare organizations in the country.

Griffith determined that these organizations met and exceeded the Baldrige criteria through

- a strong emphasis on mission, vision, and values;
- responsive leadership and worker engagement;
- disciplined strategic planning and execution;
- patient, customer, and healthcare market knowledge management;
- measurement, analysis, and improvement of performance; and
- a focus on workforce, which creates stable and enthusiastic employees.

The Baldrige Award winners demonstrate that by having an entire organization committed to quality, outstanding results can be achieved. It is also clear that the organizations that have won the Baldrige Award have developed systems to effectively execute their strategies and embed change.

The Baldrige performance criteria outline the elements a high performance organization must possess, but not how systems and structures are developed to meet these criteria. In contrast, this book provides a number of mechanisms that an organization can use to meet the criteria. Exhibit 12.2 is a graphic representation of the relationship of the chapters in this book to the Baldrige criteria.

An Action Plan for Developing an Integrated System for Execution

This integrated system for execution is designed for all sizes of healthcare delivery organizations. As has been shown throughout the preceding chapters, it is based on fundamental research, contemporary business practices from leading companies, and state-of-the-art examples from some of the best-performing healthcare systems in the United States. This integrated system can be used by medical practices (even small groups), hospitals, healthcare systems, long-term care facilities, and many other direct providers of healthcare.

Many organizations have some, but not all, of the elements of this system in place today. The following action plan can be used to move toward an integrated system for execution.

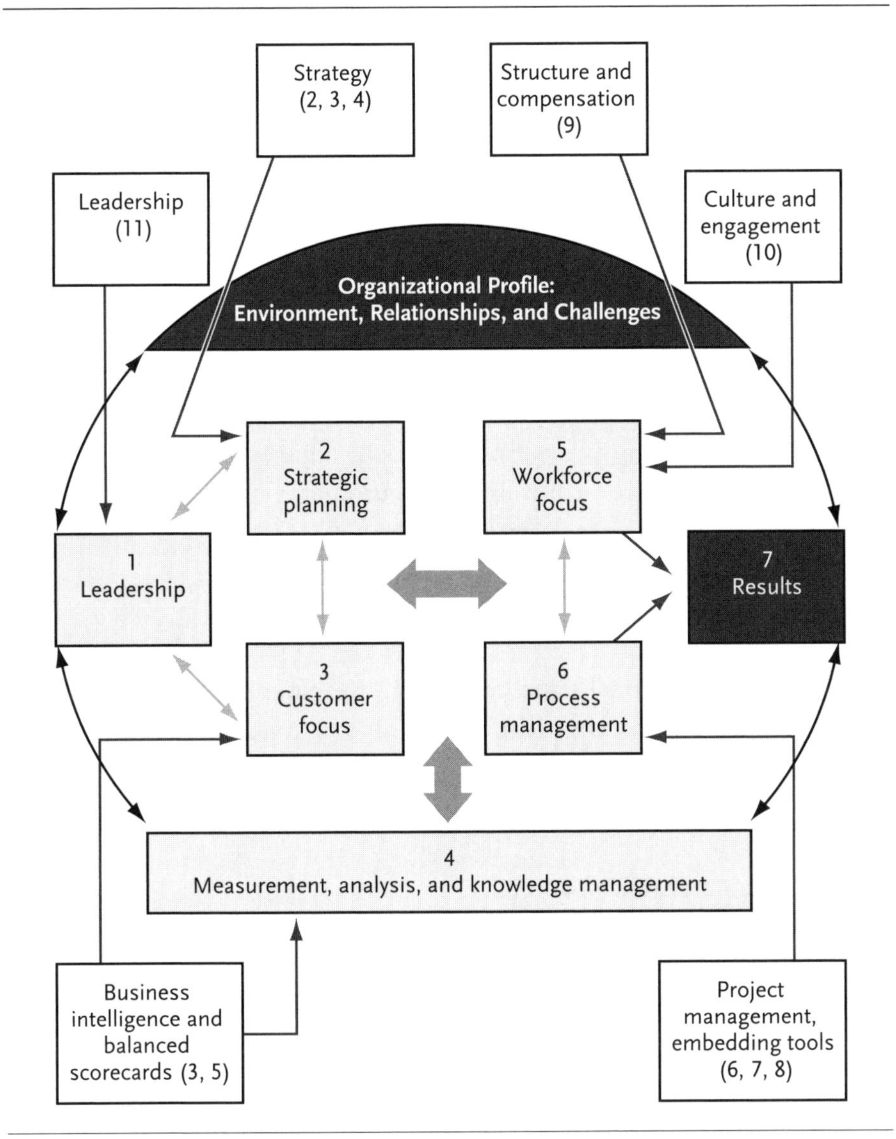

Exhibit 12.2 Baldrige Criteria and the Integrated Execution System (chapters indicated)

Strategy

1. Determine your strategy development process and consider including an approach that integrates all of the planning schools: Design, Planning, Positioning, and Learning.
2. Implement a data warehouse and do performance reporting, benchmarking, and data mining to support and refine the strategic plan.
3. Review your strategy to ensure that it has quantitative goals and metrics.
4. Test aspects of your strategic plan with scenario analysis.

5. Develop a balanced scorecard and strategy map.
6. Implement transparent scorecards at all levels of the organization.
7. Implement a periodic strategy review cycle. Keep it disconnected from operational problem solving.
8. Charter projects based on the strategy map and use the appropriate project management approach: formal PMI, Agile, Lean Six Sigma, or IHI.
9. Implement a project management office. Consider hiring PMPs[1] from industry or help existing employees achieve this certification.
10. Implement or improve systems to embed change—SOPs, process diagrams, checklists, control charts, and automated business rules and clinical decision support systems.

People

11. Review organizational structures to minimize middle management; develop employee accountability systems that maximize horizontal collaboration and reduce silo mentalities.
12. Install pay-for-performance systems that use transparent and accurate metrics.
13. Implement a physician compact.
14. Engage a consultant to review the organization's culture and improve the organization's "underlying assumptions."
15. Conduct an employee engagement survey and act on its results.
16. Understand your senior managers' leadership approaches and coach as needed.
17. Participate in adaptive and servant leadership training that emphasizes physician leadership skills.
18. Research the Baldrige criteria, make improvements, and apply for the Baldrige Award.

SUMMARY

For effective execution, an integrated system of strategy development, business tools, and people skills are needed. An organization that has implemented such a system can succeed even in chaotic environments or when unexpected events occur.

A goal for most healthcare organizations should be to meet the Baldrige criteria for performance excellence and, in some cases, make formal application. Use of the tools and methods described in this book is crucial to this endeavor.

The execution system presented in this book is comprehensive but can be implemented by most competent management teams. A set of 18 actions will launch the implementation process.

The best healthcare organizations execute crisply and effectively. Execution is about making things happen. Start today.

NOTE

1. PMP is the certification of Project Management Professional from the Project Management Institute.

HEALTHPARTNERS

Founded in 1957 as a cooperative, HealthPartners is an integrated healthcare organization providing healthcare services, health plan financing and administration, medical education, and research. It is the largest consumer-governed, nonprofit healthcare organization in the nation. The HealthPartners health plan serves 1.25 million medical and dental health plan members nationwide. It is one of the largest open access networks in the region with more than 36,000 providers and 200 hospitals and a national network of more than 650,000 providers and 6,000 hospitals. HealthPartners Medical Group includes 700 physicians, 25 primary care clinics, 9 specialty care clinics, 8 urgent care clinics, 17 pharmacies, 6 eye care centers, Integrated Home Care, and Hospice of the Lakes.

Web site: http://healthpartners.com

SMDC

St Mary's/Duluth Clinic (SMDC) Health System, a member of Essentia Health, serves a regional population of 460,000 in northeastern Minnesota, northwestern Wisconsin, and Michigan's Upper Peninsula. The integrated health system has four fully owned hospitals including St. Mary's Medical

Center, SMDC Medical Center, St. Mary's Hospital of Superior, and Pine Medical Center. In addition, it has one integrated partner, Rainy Lake Medical Center, and works in cooperation with community hospitals across the region. SMDC also includes the Duluth Clinic, a nationally recognized 400+ physician multi-specialty group, representing 55 medical specialties and providing care at 17 locations.

Web site: http://www.smdc.org/

MARSHFIELD CLINIC

When six Marshfield physicians pooled their medical expertise in 1916 to form Marshfield Clinic, they built the foundation for what has grown to become one of the largest private, multispecialty group practices in the United States. With 775 physicians in 80 medical specialties and subspecialties located in 48 locations throughout northern, central, and western Wisconsin, Marshfield Clinic's community embraces nearly all of Wisconsin and much of Michigan's Upper Peninsula.

Web site: http://www.marshfieldclinic.org

TWIN CITIES ORTHOPEDICS

Twin Cities Orthopedics (TCO) provides care to individuals of all ages with musculoskeletal injuries and conditions. TCO's 79 physicians provide diagnosis, treatment, rehabilitation, and prevention services. TCO has 30 clinics located throughout the Twin Cities.

Web site: http://www.tcomn.com/

References

Amarasingham, R., L. Plantinga, M. Diener-West, D. Gaskin, and N. Powe. 2009. "Clinical Information Technologies and Inpatient Outcomes: A Multiple Hospital Study." *Archives of Internal Medicine* 169 (2): 108–14.

American Hospital Association, Society for Healthcare Strategy and Market Development, American College of Healthcare Executives, and VHA. 2010. *Futurescan: Healthcare Trends and Implications 2010–2015*. Chicago: Health Administration Press.

Ayers, I. 2007. *Supercrunchers: Why Thinking by Numbers Is the New Way to Be Smart*. New York: Bantam Books.

Bakhtiari, E. 2010. *Five Strategies that Prove Healthcare Is Still a Growth Industry*. [Online information; retrieved 7/19/10.] www.healthleadersmedia.com/page-1/MAG-244625/Five-Strategies-that-Prove-Healthcare-is-Still-a-Growth-Industry##.

Balas, E. A., and S. A. Boren. 2000. "Managing Clinical Knowledge for Health Care Improvement." In *Yearbook of Medical Informatics 2000*, edited by J. Bemmel and A. T. McCray, 65–70. Stuttgart, Germany: Schattauer Verlagsgesellschaft.

Baldrige National Quality Program. 2010. *Health Care Criteria for Performance Excellence*. [Online information.] www.baldrige.nist.gov/HealthCare_Criteria.htm.

Bertsimas, D., M. V. Bjarnadottir, M. A. Kane, J. C. Kryder, R. Pandey, S. Vempala, and G. Wang. 2008. "Algorithmic Prediction of Health-Care Costs." *Operations Research* 56 (6): 1382.

Carden, L., and T. Egan. 2008. "Does our Literature Support Sectors Newer to Project Management? The Search for Quality Publications Relevant to Nontraditional Industries." *Project Management Journal* 39 (3): 6.

Centers for Medicare and Medicaid Services. 2009. "Medicare Acute Care Episode (ACE) Demonstration." [Online information.] www.cms.hhs.gov/DemoProjectsEvalRpts/MD/itemdetail.asp?itemID=CMS1204388.

The Commonwealth Fund Commission on a High Performance Health System. 2007. "A High Performance Health System for the United States: An Ambitious Agenda for the Next President." Washington, D.C.: The Commonwealth Fund.

Davenport, T. H., and J. G. Harris. 2007. *Competing on Analytics, The New Science of Winning*. Boston: Harvard Business School Press.

Eddy, D. M. 2007. "Linking Electronic Medical Records to Large-Scale Simulation Models: Can We Put Rapid Learning on Turbo?" *Health Affairs* 26: w125.

Englund, R. L., R. J. Graham, and P. C. Dinsmore. 2003. *Creating the Project Office—A Managers Guide to Leading Organizational Change.* San Francisco: Jossey Bass.

Etheredge, L. M. 2007. "A Rapid-Learning Health System." *Health Affairs* 26: w107.

Feltenberger, G. S., and D. N. Gans. 2008. *Benchmarking Success: The Essential Guide for Group Practices.* Englewood, CO: Medical Group Management Association.

Gawande, A. 2007. "The Checklist: If Something so Simple Can Transform Intensive Care, What Else Can It Do." *New Yorker* December 10.

Glaser, J., and J. Stone. 2008. "Effective Use of Business Intelligence." *hfm* 62 (2): 68.

Griffith, J. R. 2009. "Finding the Frontier of Hospital Management." *Journal of Healthcare Management* 54 (1): 57–72.

Haudan, J. 2008. *The Art of Engagement.* New York: McGraw Hill.

Health Information Management Systems Society (HIMSS). 2009. HIMSS Analytics. [Online information.] www.himssanalytics.org/docs/HA_EMRAM_Overview_ENG.pdf

Heifetz, R. A., and M. Linsky. 2002. *Leadership on the Line: Staying Alive Through the Dangers of Leading.* Boston: Harvard Business School Press.

Howson, C. 2008. *Successful Business Intelligence: Secrets to Making BI a Killer App.* New York: McGraw Hill.

Ingenix. 2009. Customized Fee Analyzer. [Online information; accessed 7/19/10.] http://www.shopingenix.com/upload/pdf/1626/CFA.pdf.

Institute for Healthcare Improvement. 2009. "Pursuing Perfection: The Journey to Organizational Transformation: An Interview with Mary Brainerd, CEO, HealthPartners Medical Group and Clinics." [Online article; retrieved 10/26/09.] www.ihi.org/IHI/Topics/Improvement/ ImprovementMethods/ImprovementStories/TheJourneytoOrganizationalTransformation AnInterviewwithMaryBrainerdCEOHealthPartnersMedicalGroupandC.htm.

———. 2006. "100,000 Lives Campaign." [Online information; retrieved 9/1/06.] http://www.ihi.org/IHI/Programs/Campaign/.

Kaplan, R. S., and D. P. Norton. 2008. "Mastering the Management System." *Harvard Business Review* 86 (1): 62.

———. 2001. *The Strategy-Focused Organization: How Balanced Scorecard Companies Thrive in the New Business Environment.* Boston: Harvard Business School Press.

———. 1996. *The Balanced Scorecard—Translating Strategy into Action.* Boston: Harvard Business School Press.

Kates, A., and J. R. Galbraith. 2007. *Designing Your Organization: Use the Star Model to Solve 5 Critical Design Challenges.* San Francisco: Jossey-Bass.

Keith, K. M. 2001. *The Case for Servant Leadership.* Westfield, IN: The Greenleaf Center for Servant Leadership.

Kerzner, H. 2009. *Project Management—A Systems Appoach to Planning, Scheduling and Controlling,* Third ed. New York: Wiley.

Kirby, S., and B. Robertson. 2009. "Start Small and Build Toward Business Intelligence." *hfm* 63 (1): 96.

Kroch, E., T. Vaughn, M. Koepke, S. Roman, D. Foster, S. Sinha, and S. Levey. 2006. "Hospital Boards and Quality Dashboards." *Jourrnal of Patient Safety* 2 (1): 10-19.

Letavec, C. J. 2006. *The Program Management Office—Establishing, Managing and Growing the Value of a PMO*. Fort Lauderdale, FL: J Ross Publishing.

Lewis, J. P. 2000. *The Project Manager's Desk Reference*, Second ed. Boston: McGraw Hill.

Linden, A., and J. Adler-Milstein. 2008. "Medicare Disease Management in Policy Context." *Health Care Financing Review* 29 (3): 1.

Lindgren, M., and H. Bandhold. 2009. *Scenario Planning: The Link Between Future and Strategy*. New York: Palgrave–Macmillan.

Macey, W. H., B. Schneider, K. M. Barbera, and S. A. Young. 2009. *Employee Engagement: Tools for Analysis, Practice and Competitive Advantage*. Malden, MA: Wiley Blackwell.

Microsoft Office Project Professional. 2003. Help Screens.

Milstein, A., and E. Gilbertson. 2009. "American Medical Home Runs." *Health Affairs* 28 (5): 1317.

Mintzberg, H., B. Ahlstrand, and J. Lampel. 1998. *Strategy Safari: A Guided Tour Through the Wilds of Strategic Management*. New York: Free Press (Simon and Schuster).

Mountford J., and C. Webb. 2009. "When Clinicians Lead." [Online article.] *McKinsey Quarterly* http://mkqpreview1.qdweb.net/Health_Care/Strategy_Analysis/When_clinicians_lead_2293.

National Institute of Standards and Technology. 2009. "The Quest for Excellence—Poudre Valley Health System: Malcolm Baldrige National Quality Award for 2008." www.baldrige.nist.gov.

Niven, P. R. 2005. *Balanced Scorecard Diagnostics: Maintaining Maximum Performance*. New York: Wiley.

———. 2002. *Balanced Scorecard Step by Step: Maximizing Performance and Maintaining Results*. New York: Wiley.

Project Management Institute. 2008. *A Guide to the Project Management Body of Knowledge*, Fourth ed. Newtown Square, PA: Project Management Institute.

Reinertsen, J., M. Bisognano, and M. Pugh. 2008. *Seven Leadership Leverage Points for Organization-Level Improvement in Health Care*. Cambridge, MA: Insititute for Healthcare Improvement.

Roberts, J. 2004. *The Modern Firm: Organizational Design for Performance and Growth*. New York: Oxford University Press.

Ruud, K., M. Johnson, C. Schinstock, J. Liesinger, and J. Naessens. 2008. *Accuracy of Text Mining in Identifying Follow-up Appointment Criteria from Hospital Discharge Records*. Rochester, MN: Mayo Clinic Study.

Schein, E. H. 2004. *Organizational Culture and Leadership*, Third ed. Hoboken, NJ: Jossey-Bass.

Schultz, E. 2009. "Future of Healthcare." Presentation at the University of St. Thomas, November.

Senge, P. M. 1990. *The Fifth Discipline: The Art and Practice of the Learning Organization*. New York: Doubleday.

Silver, M., T. Sakata, H. C. Su, C. Herman, S. B. Dolins, and M. J. O'Shea. 2001. "Case Study: How to Apply Data Mining Techniques in a Healthcare Data Warehouse." *Journal of Healthcare Information Management* 15 (2): 155–64.

Stoller, J. K. 2008. "Developing Physician-Leaders: Key Competencies and Available Programs." *The Journal of Health Administration Education* 25 (4): 307–28.

Turban, E., R. Sharda, J. E. Aronson, and D. King. 2008. *Business Intelligence: A Managerial Approach.* Upper Saddle River, NJ: Pearson Prentice Hall.

Wang, X. S., L. Nayda, and R. Dettinger. 2007. "Infrastructure for a Clinical-Decision-Intelligence System." *IBM Systems Journal* 46 (1): 151.

Zuckerman, A. M. 2005. *Healthcare Strategic Planning*, Second ed. Chicago: Health Adminstration Press.

Index

Communication: during clinical change process, 110; face-to-face, 104, 125, 129

Communication plans, in project management, 73, 93

Communication skills, of leaders, 166

Compacts, 140, 141–143, 178

Compensation: compacts for, 140, 141–143; effective systems of, 138–139; pay-for-performance systems of, 178; professional services agreement (PSA) model of, 139–143; variable, 143

Competency, scenario analysis of, 44

Competitiveness, 138

Complementarity, 44, 137

Conflict, adaptive change-related, 162–163

Conflict management, team approach in, 164

Contemplative analysis, 24

Contracts, differentiated from compacts, 140

Control charts, 119, 120

Cooperation, *versus* initiative, 137

Cost reimbursement contracts, 96

Crossing the Quality Chasm (Institute of Medicine), 1

Cultural change, relationship to physician leadership, 165

Culture, organizational, 4–5, 145–158; artifact level of, 146, 147, 148, 155–156; case examples of, 153–157; definition of, 145–146; development of, 146; elements of, 145–146, 147; espoused beliefs and values level of, 146, 147, 155–156; iceberg metaphor of, 146, 147; implication for project management, 77; relationship to employee engagement, 149–157; shaping and embedding of, 148; underlying assumptions level of, 146–148, 155, 156–157, 178

Current procedural terminology (CPT) codes, 31–32

Customer perspective, on organizational performance, 55, 56, 57–58, 69

Customer satisfaction, agile project management approach to, 104

Customer structure, 134, 135, 136, 143

D

Daily huddle meetings, 113, 124, 129

Dashboards, 25, 26, 54, 119–121; graphical data displays of, 119, 120, 129; for organizational culture management, 155; for preventive services, 126, 128

Data access, 24–25

Data analysis, 23–24

Data collection: for balanced scorecards, 63; in strategic planning, 19–23

Data displays: of benchmark data, 34, 119, 120, 121; graphical, 25–29, 119, 120, 129

Data marts, 22, 23

Data mining, 20, 23, 29–31; association in, 30–31; case examples of, 35–37; classification in, 30–31; cluster analysis in, 30–31; definition of, 29; text mining, 31, 35–36; Web mining, 31

Data warehousing, 20, 21–23, 177; case examples of, 34, 35, 37; comparison with transactional data systems, 24; data access in, 24–25; erroneous data entry in, 23;

extract, transform, and load (ETL) component of, 22, 23, 34, 37, 38; in integrated healthcare systems, 173; of metadata, 23

Dean Health System, benchmarking use by, 34–35

Denver International Airport, 72

Design, organizational. *See* Structure, organizational

Design School model, of strategic planning, 10, 13, 18, 50, 56, 177

Detailed task scheduling, 108

Diagnosis-related groups (DRGs), 49–50

DMAIC framework, 105–106, 108, 109, 114

Doughnut charts, 27, 28

Drill-down reporting, 24, 25, 35, 119

Drug prescriptions, 35

E

Eddy, David, 111

Effectiveness, scenario analysis of, 44

Electronic health records (EHRs): data warehousing of, 20, 21–23; definition of, 39; HIMSS Analytics EMR Adoption Model of, 20; implementation of, 20; use in clinical research, 111

Electronic health records (EHRs) systems: clinical support function of, 122–124; text storage function of, 36

Electronic medical records (EMRs), definition of, 39

Emergent strategy formulation, 10

Emotional intelligence, 166

Empowerment, 165

Engagement, of employees: factors affecting, 4–5, 149; "line of sight" approach to, 152–153; relationship to organizational culture, 149–157; strategies for improvement of, 151–153; surveys of, 149–151, 154–155, 158, 178

Environmental assessment, 13, 14, 33

Episode of treatment groups (ETGs), 23, 37, 38

Equity, internal and external, 138

Errors, in data entry, 23

Execution, in healthcare: barriers to, 1; integrated system for, 2, 5, 173–179; need for, 1–6

Exegesis, 39

Exegetical analysis, 24, 25

External assessment, in strategic plan development, 19–21

Extract, transform, and load (ETL) component, of data warehousing, 22, 23, 34, 37, 38

F

Feasibility analysis, of project charters, 77–78

Feedback, 115–116, 117; balancing, 116, 117, 119, 124, 129; reinforcing, 116, 117

Filtering rules, 121–122

Financial perspective, on organizational performance, 55, 56, 57–58, 69

Financial reports, as primary management tool, 53–54

Financing, of healthcare, 2, 3

Fishbone diagrams, 117

Fixed-price contracts, 96
Flowcharts, 117, 118
Force field analysis, 94
Foresight, of leaders, 165
Formulaic analysis, 24
Freedom, role in employee engagement, 149, 150
Fuel gauge indicators, of performance, 26
Functional organization structure, 133–134, 135, 143
Futurescan, 42

G

General systems theory, 115–116, 129
Globalization, 42
Goals: of high-performance healthcare systems, 1; "line of sight" approach to, 152–153; "stretch," 65
Graphical data displays, 25–29, 119, 120, 129
Great Society, 2, 9
Greenleaf, Robert, 163–164
Griffith, John, 175–176
Growth-share matrix, 11, 12

H

Harrah's Casino, 21
Harvard University, 160
Health Administration Press, 42
Healthcare: access to, 1; changing emphasis in, 2, 3
Healthcare Effectiveness Data and Information set (HEDIS) measures, 111
Healthcare Information and Management Systems Society (HIMSS), electronic medical record implementation model of, 20
Healthcare Operations Management (McLaughlin and Hays), 29, 55, 58, 80–81, 94, 95, 104
Healthcare policy, 1
Healthcare Strategic Planning (Zuckerman), 13
Healthcare systems, high-performance, 1–2, 5
HealthPartners, 13, 15; business intelligence system of, 34; Care, Innovation, and Measurement department of, 111–112; organizational culture change strategy of, 153–154
Heifetz, Ron, 160, 161–163
HIMSS Analytics EMR Adoption Model, 20
Histograms, 117
"Holding environment," for conflict management, 162–163
Hospital performance metrics, 32
Huddles, 113, 124, 129

I

"If-then" statements, 59, 60, 62
Implementation planning, 13, 14
Incremental strategy formulation, 10
Information systems, 19; of project management offices, 100
Information technology (IT), vendor contracts for, 77
Information technology (IT) departments, 121

Initiative(s): *versus* cooperation, 137; development of, 59; failure of, 64; implementation of, 62; linkage of, 62–63; measures for, 59, 60; for organizational synergy, 62; prioritization of, 65; strategy maps of, 60–62; targets of, 63, 65, 69
Innovation. *See* Clinical innovation
Institute for Healthcare Improvement (IHI), 154; "Hospital to Home strategy of, 18; improvement map of, 110, 114; leadership model of, 166–167; "100,000 Lives" campaign of, 110; project improvement model of, 106–107, 108, 109
Institute of Medicine (IOM), *Crossing the Quality Chasm,* 1
Integrated system, for execution in healthcare: action plan for, 176–178; demand for, 2; implementation of, 173–179; leader of, 178; Malcolm Baldrige Award criteria for, 175–176, 177, 178, 179
Integrative roles, 136
Internal business process perspective, on organizational performance, 56, 57–58, 69
Internal performance analysis, 38; data access in, 24–25; data analysis in, 23–24; data collection for, 19–23; data displays in, 25–29; of data sources, 19–21

J

Johns Hopkins Hospital, 118
Joint Commission, 33

K

Kaizen events, 106
Kaplan, Robert, 54–55, 64
Knowledge transfer, among colleagues, 125

L

Lagging indicators. *See* Outcome indicators
Leaders, role in organizational culture, 148, 157
Leadership, 159–170; adaptive, 5, 160–163, 167–169, 178; danger of, 160–161; "great man" theory of, 160; Institute for Healthcare Improvement model of, 166–167; of integrated healthcare systems, 178; as performance criterion, 175, 176, 177; physician, 165–166; power-based, 164; relationship to organizational culture, 153; servant, 163–165, 169–170, 178; team approach in, 164
Leadership skills, training in, 165–166
Leading indicators. *See* Performance drivers
Lean process improvement approach, 58, 104
Lean Six Sigma process improvement approach, 104–106, 137; DMAIC framework of, 104–106, 108, 109, 114
Leapfrog group, 33
Learning perspective, on organizational performance, 56, 57–58, 69
Learning School model, of strategic planning, 11–12, 15, 16, 50, 56, 175, 177
Lindgren, Mats, 42
Line charts, 26
Linsky, Marty, 160
Listening skills, of leaders, 161–162, 164

U

Uncertainty, of trends, 43–44
Unexpected events, response to, 174–175
United States Department of Commerce, 175–176, 177
United States Department of Defense, 72
United States Preventive Services Task Force, 110, 114
University of Michigan, 175
University of St. Thomas, Physician Leadership College, 5, 159

V

Vanderbilt Medical Center, clinical decision support system of, 125–126, 127
Vendors: contracts with, 96–98; of employee engagement surveys, 149–150; procurement of, 95–96, 97

Vincent Valley Healthcare, 5, 15–17; accountable care organization (ACO) project of, 112–113, 167–169; data warehousing use by, 37; medical home project of, 45–47, 126, 128, 157, 169–170; Medicare acute care episode (ACE) project of, 82–101, 155–157; preventive services dashboard of, 126, 128; professional services agreement of, 140, 142–143; project management office of, 101, 113; project management process of, 71–101; scenario analysis use at, 45–50; strategy maps of, 67–68

W

Washington, George, 164
Web mining, 31
Work, technical *versus* adaptive, 160
Workforce, engaged, 149; surveys of, 149–151

ABOUT THE AUTHOR

DANIEL MCLAUGHLIN

Daniel McLaughlin, MHA, is director of the Center for Health and Medical Affairs in the Opus College of Business at the University of St. Thomas. Prior to this position, he was executive director of the National Institute of Health Policy at the University of St. Thomas. From 1984 to 1992, Mr. McLaughlin was CEO of Hennepin County Medical Center and director of the county health system.

Mr. McLaughlin has served as chair of the National Association of Public Hospitals and Health Systems. He served on President Clinton's Task Force on Health Care Reform in 1993. He holds degrees in electrical engineering and healthcare administration from the University of Minnesota. In addition to his administrative responsibilities, Mr. McLaughlin is active in teaching and research at the University of St. Thomas, with emphasis on healthcare operations, leadership, and policy.

He is also the author of *Healthcare Operations Management* and *Responding to Healthcare Reform*, both published by Health Administration Press.